The

Cholesterol

Trap!

Re-Examining your Doctor's Prescription

Dr. Dorothy Adamiak, ND

LiveUthing Press

ISBN-13: 978-1541247734
ISBN-10: 1541247736

Disclaimer

All information provided in this book is for educational purposes only. The information is not intended as a substitute for the medical advice of physicians. The reader should regularly consult a physician in matters relating to his/her health and particularly with respect to any symptoms that may require diagnosis or medical attention. This information is not intended to replace clinical judgment or guide individual patient care in any manner.

Use of this book implies your acceptance of this disclaimer.

Contents

Chapter 1

The uphill battle against cholesterol

Oops! Your recent physical did not go that well. You have high cholesterol.

The results weren't a big surprise. Heart disease runs in your family. Your dad just had a stroke and had hard time with recovery. Your mom has been battling erratic blood pressure, which only got worse after dad landed in the hospital. Hmmm… if only you did not have that extra bacon slice and a shot of whiskey last Saturday the results could have been different. Maybe cholesterol would not go up and you would be just fine.

But that was just one fun day. Otherwise you were very careful with your menu. You followed a low-fat diet that was supposed to keep cholesterol down.

Nobody likes dieting, definitely not you, but the thought of getting heart disease sent chills down your spine. The horrifying possibility made you stick to Cheerios and bananas. Low-fat diet was meant to keep cholesterol at bay. It was supposed to counteract your body's natural tendency to build it up. But a low grease menu did not do what you were hoping for. Tuna salads and baby carrots did not make an iota of difference.

The doctor was right. One cannot escape heart disease and you are a living proof. Heart disease is hereditary and high cholesterol is inevitable at a certain age. It is just a matter of time. And now the genetic destiny is catching up with you.

Your doctor says that at this point there is not much you can do except filling out his prescription. Maybe he is right. Maybe cholesterol-lowering medication is the surest way to prevent heart disease. The first hundred pages on Google, your favorite TV host, and your neighbour, a registered nurse, all share your doctor's opinion.

Chapter 2

Cholesterol myths are hard to die

Prevention and treatment of heart disease has been infiltrated by many myths. From cholesterol tests to cholesterol advice we continue being fed misinformation. Even top doctors are not spared from repeating the common myths. Many still believe that avoiding eggs, eating margarine and taking daily meds is the best prescription for health, despite research proving that low-cholesterol diets don`t work and meds have more side effects than benefits.

Cholesterol fantasies don`t want to die and they are the number one reason for our health failures. Did you know that despite massive medical and dietary efforts, our hearts are not any better off than they were a hundred years ago?

In early 1900s when we were gobbling fats without a second thought and heart meds weren`t discovered yet, we had just a fraction of the cardiovascular deaths that we currently have.[1] Today we have more heart-related deaths than a century ago despite all modern life conveniences, abundance of food, swift transportation, internet communication, specialized medical training, access to countless clinics and hospitals, extensive prevention programs, early detection policies, advanced high-tech diagnostics, and shelves full of drugs. Something is really wrong.

Cholesterol myths are widespread. You likely have fallen for them as well, so has George who shuns red meat, John that has eggs only once a week, Jane that follows Pritikin`s diet, and Mia that orders skim milk smoothies. These are your internet buddies, real friends, neighbours, co-workers, and beloved celebrities.

The cholesterol phobia is not limited to non-experts. It infiltrates health clinics as well. Ask your physician's secretary or the physician himself next time around. You will be amazed how many people have a fear of cholesterol and firmly believe that high cholesterol is the cause of heart disease and fat avoidance is the key.

There are many cholesterol myths that get passed around. Among the most harmful ones are:

- Heart disease is genetic
- Heart disease is irreversible
- High cholesterol causes heart disease
- High cholesterol blocks arteries
- Lowering cholesterol prevents heart disease

And finally the most perpetuated cholesterol myths of all:

- Dietary cholesterol leads to heart disease, and
- Low fat diet keeps the heart healthy

Should we then continue living in fear while nervously picking grease off the plate? Should we look at our lab results in terror only to faithfully line up in pharmacies to fill life-saving prescriptions?

Over many years of clinical practice I noticed a very dangerous trend. Exactly those patients who were careful about their diets and took cholesterol-lowering drugs scored the lowest in health. One would think that they should be the healthiest of all the patients, but the opposite was actually true. They were the most ailment-riddled, achy, stiff, and overweight. They were in stark contrast to flourishing and robust patients that did not care to please their doctors with desirable behavior.

Such incredible disparity between these two types of patients was hard not to notice. It was also the very reason why I wrote this book. I could no longer ignore that existing huge gap between what we believe should happen vs. what actually happens when we do certain things. Heart disease is not only preventable. It is completely reversible. But, we cannot achieve it by lowering cholesterol or following a low fat diet.

Chapter 3

Heart disease today

Who isn't afraid of heart disease? Heart disease is so widespread that without any doubt you know someone who already has it. From high blood pressure, to atherosclerosis and stroke... heart disease can manifest in many different ways.

Your doctor is not exaggerating. Heart disease is not the same as stomach flu, sprained ankle, or acne. Unlike those trivial maladies, heart disease is serious. It steals lives and it does so on a massive scale. It is responsible for bigger things than a minor diarrhea, a limp, or a pimple. Heart disease is heartless. It causes awful tragedies, crippling disabilities and cruel deaths.

Heart disease is a 20th century phenomenon. It is hard to believe but we were not affected by it in the past. While unheard of in early 1900s heart disease suddenly surfaced after the 2nd World War. It peaked between 1960s and 1990s. Now 30 years later despite billions of dollars spent on prevention and treatment we are still under its dark spell.

Heart disease continues to be a monumental concern. Despite six decades of the war on cholesterol the list of the cardiac fatalities remains very long. Today even with massive educational and pharmaceutical effort, heart disease kills more than half a million Americans a year. It continues to be the biggest health scare for modern man.

- Heart disease is the number one cause of death in the United States[2]
- One in three deaths in North America is due to a heart-related causes
- About 610,000 Americans die of heart disease every year[3]
- Every 43 seconds someone in America gets diagnosed with heart disease
- Every 40 seconds someone in America dies of it

Did you know that cardiovascular diseases claim more lives than all forms of cancer combined? While the most feared breast cancer takes 40,000 lives a year, heart disease takes fifteen times that many.

Did you know that 735,000 people in the USA have heart attacks each year and 120,000 of those die?[4] It is like every single person in Seattle, WA gets a heart attack and one in six dies from it.

Did you know that blocked arteries account for even more fatalities than heart attacks? In 2008 alone coronary artery disease was blamed for 405,309 deaths in USA,[5] which is more or less the entire population of Oakland, California.

The cost of the epidemic is enormous. Estimated annual economic burden for the USA is $313 billion. Although the average taxpayer can't tell how much of their hard earned money goes towards this burden I may illustrate the financial impact differently.

To pay in full for the economic impact of heart disease every single US resident, including infants and veterans, must contribute $1,000 annually towards this cause. To put it yet in other words, heart disease is so costly that it can sink six million US households into stark poverty. If we spread the burden over 6 million families each would have to pay US $50,000 annually to bear the soaring costs.

Where is this US $313 billion going? 121 billion goes for direct health care costs such as doctors, clinical procedures and medication. The remaining 192 billion[6,7] is associated with productivity loss and work absenteeism. This is the indirect cost that pertains to inability to perform the duties due to illness.

With high cost and no real solution in sight heart disease continues to be a hot topic. But headlines do not exaggerate the rate and extent of the problem. Everyone is at risk. Not because heart disease is hereditary, but because many people carry at least one factor that predisposes them to falling pray to it.

Obesity and high blood pressure are the front runners. They are followed by a few other well-acknowledged risk factors. Five are listed below. The percentages refer to the proportion of people influenced by the respective factors.

- obesity, about 74%[8]
- high blood pressure, about 30%[9]
- high cholesterol, about 30%[10], and
- smoking, about 17%[11]
- depression, about 7%.[12]

Note that high cholesterol is one of the risks listed for heart disease. But, cholesterol-heart disease link is not as straightforward as many people believe. Although, it is true that cholesterol and heart disease *may* go in the same direction, blaming cholesterol for heart troubles should now be considered an outdated concept.

There are still many unknowns about cholesterol, but it looks like we are in the process of discovering that cholesterol may not be an enemy after all. It may be a real friend capable of warning of declining health. It is slowly becoming clearer to us that cholesterol may be a valuable health marker, a major contributor to hormonal and antioxidant reserves, and not the heart killer as seen by many people. We may be shortly coming to the conclusion that the pharmacological "correction" of cholesterol numbers is a silly concept that goes against health.

Chapter 4

A different look at cholesterol

"Know your cholesterol numbers!" We are being told that every responsible citizen should know whether they have any cardiovascular risks. Cholesterol has become the main cardiovascular screen used by virtually all medical doctors. It is simple, inexpensive, and well-studied. Thus there is not a patient that would walk out of the cardiologist's office without having his cholesterol tested.

Unlike doctors, few patients have inclination to contemplate their blood work. Medicine is complicated and that's why patients rely on their physicians to guide them towards better health. Patients seldom look at their own lab results, because they feel they won't be able to understand it. Studies show that 90% of people don't know their blood pressure numbers. Cholesterol numbers are even more intimidating.

"High cholesterol" sounds scary. It freezes people into panic. But it is exactly this reaction that backfires on us. Hysteria wins. Patients desperately scramble to lower their cholesterol without any understanding what it actually means. Few muster the courage to ask questions, check their own lab numbers or look for solutions beyond drugs and supplements. Once "high cholesterol" is announced, worry overshadows all logic.

Fear transforms "high cholesterol" into a horrifying image of blocked arteries, strokes and heart attacks. Fear shapes cholesterol into a monster that can barricade blood flow at any time, a ruthless heart exterminator that is looking out for its next prey. This yellow artery plugging beast can be highly dangerous and we need to chase it out of the body.

Relax! Let's step back a little bit.

What does "cholesterol" mean to you? If you say: heart disease, plugged arteries, heart attack, stroke, disability, and death, you are not alone. That's exactly what all my patients said when I asked them this question. Cholesterol has been demonized so badly and so consistently that by now everyone sees cholesterol as a mean hearted overlord.

Absolutely every one of those who answered my question believed that cholesterol was bad. No one said anything good. No one mentioned that cholesterol had anything to do with strength, youthfulness, glowing skin and robustness. Not a single man knew that cholesterol was needed to get an erection. Not a single student or pregnant woman knew that cholesterol was needed for a normal brain function.

Years of badmouthing cholesterol has paid off. Today few consider that cholesterol may not only be good, but also necessary. Few know that cholesterol is absolutely vital for life and that it constitutes a basis for health. Few are aware that without cholesterol we would not even be alive.

Think about it for a moment. Unless Mother Nature is into cardiovascular mockery why would it let our bodies make a substance that is supposed to kill us all? Unless the liver develops a deep-seated aversion towards the heart, why would it pump the yellow goo that is to slam shut its arteries? Is there some kind of genetic vessel clogging conspiracy that researchers are yet to discover? Sort of like self-destructive behaviour humans tend to fall for?

It's silly, isn't it? Now on a serious note.

All human bodies require cholesterol. The substance is so vital that its sudden lack can halt all essential body functions in a single day. Without cholesterol all our fundamental tasks would come to a standstill: feeling, thinking, healing, growing, and even maintaining blood pressure.

Cholesterol plays various roles, some of which we already know, and many of which we are yet to identify. Despite that educational gap somebody decided some time ago that in order to be healthier we need to suppress it. A few decades later we start scratching our heads as researchers and doctors are realizing that lowering the numbers may be futile and quite frankly foolish. Cholesterol is too deeply interwoven in cellular health to be treated in isolation. We cannot simply lower it and expect zero health implications.

Cholesterol makes membranes

Every human cell is dressed in a jacket called membrane. Just as jackets have buttons, membranes have cholesterol. Cholesterol is an integral part of the protective coat of the cell and it isn't there for fashion. It is there on purpose.

The buttons that open and close the jacket regulate air flow. They decide whether you will feel hot and cold, sweaty and uncomfortable, or breezy and fresh. Cholesterol sort of does that as well. It directs information flow, prevents signal gridlock, and allows for transport of goods to and from the cells. Similarly to buttons that regulate the jacket penetrability, cholesterol regulates membrane fluidity and permeability. Without cholesterol, membranes lose their function and the cellular coat becomes useless.

Researchers agree that cells cannot work without cholesterol. It is too important. It provides structural support and decides on what cells can do. When membranes are deprived of cholesterol, cellular functions can get completely crippled and come to a standstill.[13]

Cholesterol makes hormones

Bricks build houses. Cholesterol builds hormones. Hormones are complex molecules. They are not like single atom minerals, iron or potassium. They are much more complicated. They are made of diverse parts which may include strings of proteins or beads of cholesterol.

Not all hormones need cholesterol, but steroids definitely do. Steroids are derived from cholesterol. Thus all steroid hormones such as cortisol, growth hormone, testosterone, progesterone, or estrogen need cholesterol for their production.

What happens if the body does not have cholesterol? In such a case the body can't make steroids and the consequences are daring. Depending which hormone is missing a person may end up with congestive heart failure, diabetes, or dwarfishness. In less dramatic cases one may have to live with joint pains, erectile dysfunction, or infertility.

Steroids are extremely important. They regulate many body systems and their role is especially pronounced in water balance, stress response and sexual development. They decide on the body aesthetics, recovery time from an illness, and annual physical lab results. They decide on biceps size, intensity of inflammation, and blood pressure numbers. Steroids regulate our bodily functions and cholesterol allows them to exist.

Cholesterol makes vitamin D

Did you know that vitamin D is a hormone? It is also a steroid and like every other steroid it requires cholesterol for its production.

The importance of vitamin D has been highlighted by the media. Now everyone knows that lack of this vitamin could have devastating consequences. Low vitamin D is linked to development of numerous chronic problems including cardiovascular and immune system compromise. Its insufficiency leads to heart disease and increases cancer risk. It causes osteoporosis and magnifies the risk for bone fractures. Vitamin D is also needed for proper brain function.

Did you also know that about every second American adult is vitamin D deficient?[14] Research suggests that lowering cholesterol has something to do with it, as it directly impacts vitamin D stores. Cholesterol and vitamin D go together. People who have low cholesterol are also low in vitamin D.[15]

Cholesterol supports digestion

The liver doesn't just make cholesterol for the sake of disposing it. Cholesterol is too precious to be discarded, so the liver converts it to bile acids. These in turn help break down the food and digest lipids. Without bile acids we would not be able to make use of the nutrients that are carried by dietary fats.

Fat is home to several vital nutrients. Fat carries fat-soluble vitamins which include, besides the already mentioned vitamin D, vitamin E, A, and K. These fat-soluble vitamins are necessary for maintaining arterial health and blood flow. So indirectly bile acids, a by-product of cholesterol, help guard against cardiovascular accidents.

Vitamin E and K regulate blood thickness. They work together. One keeps the blood flow clot-free and the other prevents it from over-thinning. Vitamin E and K are also the very vitamins that prevent hardening of the arteries. Together they maintain blood vessels elasticity.

It is shocking to learn that in order to have a healthy heart we need to eat fat and that in order to absorb the vitamins we actually need to have cholesterol.

Cholesterol shelters nervous system

Nerves work similarly to electrical wires. They conduct an electrical signal via its pre-established network. Ideally the impulse goes from one end to another in the nick of time. This can happen only if the signal is adequately shielded and does not dissipate while on its way to the destination. How can the signal be protected? Electrical wires are embedded in non-conductive plastic tubes. Nerves are shielded by non-conductive fatty sheets.

Fat does not conduct electricity and it is perfectly suited for such an insulating job. Nerve fibres that are fat-wrapped are least subject to losing the signal. Fatty cholesterol is an incredible insulator. It greatly increases the speed of the signal and prevents its shorting with the neighbouring network.

Well-insulated nerves facilitate quick reflexes and speedy reactions. They boost swift thinking and effortless memorizing. Fat-submerged, cholesterol coated nerves are the best performers and that's why 25% of body cholesterol is found in the brain.[16] Research confirmed that people with lower cholesterol are more likely to lose their marbles.[17]

Chapter 5

What's behind the cholesterol scare

Cholesterol propaganda is incredibly unfair. It wrongly portrays cholesterol as a cardiovascular menace, instead of acknowledging it is a major life pillar. The hype has infiltrated medical books with horrible consequences. Few doctors grasp the importance of cholesterol in human health. Few understand that cholesterol is a health marker pointing to robustness of an individual and his lifestyle habits. Few consider advising on lifestyle changes due to their lack of expertise in this area and even fewer ponder the multiple, long-term complications, before medicating the lab test numbers.

Doctors do what doctors are taught to do and old habits are hard to break. Misinformation about cholesterol lingers due to, often purposefully, skewed medical curricula. High cholesterol continues to scare people and keep doctors prescribing "lifesaving" medication. The system works. It sells. Why should anyone strive to change the beneficiaries then?

The government appears to be the biggest perpetrator in this scheme. It is incredibly skilled at creating cholesterol panic. Government websites scaring their visitors of the dangers of high cholesterol are flourishing. For example, CDC, Centres for Disease and Control and Prevention web pages are full of cholesterol-blaming statements. Here are some examples:

- *"People with high total cholesterol have approximately twice the risk of heart disease"*
- *"Having high blood cholesterol puts you at risk of heart disease, the leading cause of death in the United States*
- *Your body needs some cholesterol, but it can build up on the walls of your arteries and lead to heart disease and stroke when you have too much in your blood*
- *The average American adult has cholesterol level of about 200 mg/dL, which is borderline high risk*
- *Lowering your cholesterol can reduce your risk of having a heart attack, needing heart bypass surgery or angioplasty, and dying of heart disease"*

The message is straightforward and the guidelines reflect that. There is no "if's" or "but's" about cholesterol. High is bad and should be feared. Total cholesterol above 200 mg/dL (5.2 mmol/l) increases the risk for heart disease and the higher the numbers the worse it gets.

The guidelines become the prevailing mantra, and once established it trickles down to medical schools, hospitals, clinics, and eventually they decide what prescription your doctor writes. They change clinicians' and patients' perception on what is safe, unsafe and needs to be done. The guidelines become the prevailing truth regardless of the reality.

Although the guidelines may raise a few concerns, few dare to question what the government dictates. Your doctor cannot challenge things either. His job is to follow the guidelines, not to create any conflict by researching on his own, changing the established protocols, and possibly putting you "at risk". Everyone knows that "bad" doctors lose their jobs. As a result, every patient is subject to routine cholesterol tests and routine cholesterol-lowering protocols whether they need them or not.

It was frustrating for me to see how the omnipotent guidelines and generalized protocols make my patients worse off rather than better. In the past I scratched my head asking the question "why isn't anybody saying anything and why is everyone eager to comply?" Then I found the answer: it's because the system is perfect. It has been well masterminded. The government defines the rules and as long as everyone conforms to them, the taxpayers get to live in peace: doctors keep their jobs, pharmacists get to sell their goods and the patient is told he is getting a healthier heart and longer life! It is win-win-win for everyone!

So what's wrong with the guidelines and the messages broadcasted by the government? I see a few flaws. The first one is "all in one bag" approach where every patient is treated in the same way. The second is the statement that high cholesterol kills.

Cholesterol is not just one substance. It is many. Cholesterol awareness is work in progress. As researchers keep on discovering its new variants we keep on learning about their different roles. No way can we say that our knowledge is complete. We are just starting. So far we have gathered bits and pieces, fragments of data, and glimpses of various effects. It would be inappropriate to make firm conclusions and sweeping statements based on the above. But it is done nonetheless.

Even though the progress is slow, we are inching forward. Few years back doctors could see only one cholesterol number on the lab reports. Today we know that different cholesterol types perform such different functions that they cannot be lumped together. Thanks to technological advancement, now doctors can look up three or more separate cholesterol types on standard lab sheets. Better reporting reflects our upgraded view of human physiology.

But reporting progress does not necessarily parallel human desire for simplicity. Although we know that fitting cholesterol under one umbrella of ugly is wrong, everybody does it. The government, the media, clinicians and dietitians are all guilty of mixing up numbers, sources and effects.

Did you notice that we have a war on cholesterol and not a war on bad cholesterol? Did you notice that everyone talks about suppressing cholesterol, not improving its ratio? Did you know that even though it is the liver that makes and regulates all the cholesterol, we are told to cut down on butter? And finally did you notice that despite the cholesterol-lowering effort heart statistics are in a dark place?

The cholesterol confusion is great and our purchasing habits reflect it. Low-fat diets, zero-cholesterol meals, and cholesterol-lowering medications have never been more popular. They fly off the shelves as we zero in on suppressing cholesterol. After all, when it comes to fats we are told that lower is better.

Strangely, even progressive labs reflect that attitude. Did you know that the range for total cholesterol has a well-defined *upper* limit to warn about the dangers of high cholesterol, but there is no *lower* limit whatsoever, as if suggesting that zero cholesterol is a desirable body state? Of course it is not. People with zero cholesterol are dead.

Even though our bodies have a physiological need for cholesterol, many doctors are in a race to reach the lowest number possible believing that cholesterol near zero constitutes a victory over heart disease. Too bad, because many of those "well-taken-care-of" patients also feel that they are at their worse state of health. Sadly, patients' complaints seldom matter. The guidelines and lab numbers come first.

Besides, health professionals are humans and just like everyone else they like to simplify things. Since it is easier to look at one number than comparing three or four, clinicians tend to look at total cholesterol and base their entire assessment on that one number. Although wrong, such lab number treatment is extremely common.

Statistically speaking, eight out of ten patients I have shared with other physicians was misinformed about their cholesterol profile. The cholesterol concerns were overestimated and only lead to unnecessary treatment. Because overzealousness of doctors is common, I advise every patient to look at the numbers personally, regardless of the clinician's opinion.

Maybe you have never seen a lab report before and maybe getting the first glimpse of it may sound scary. But you don't need to have a master's degree to read cholesterol numbers. All you need to do is locate the word cholesterol on the report. Once you have done that, look around and locate two abbreviations:

- HDL – this is your good cholesterol (this one reflects your robustness)
- LDL – this is your "bad" cholesterol (no cholesterol is bad, this is just its popular nickname)

The numbers slightly to the right of these abbreviations are your results. Disregard anything else and don't worry about the ranges for now. All you should care for is that you have heaps of HDL, and some LDL.

Disregard your total cholesterol number entirely. It is irrelevant. Your job is *not* to decrease *total* cholesterol, but to improve LDL/HDL ratio. For most people that would mean increasing HDL and decreasing LDL.

Ideally you would see that HDL equals or exceeds LDL. Don't fret if you don't have that. Perfect proportions are rare to find. These would reflect outstanding health. But for many reasons perfect health in North America is very rare.

The most common scenario is that HDL is half or one third of LDL. That's not good. Bringing HDL and LDL closer together is possible, but requires substantial lifestyle effort. This is exactly why so many people prefer pills.

Before you reach for your doctor's prescription know that in order to improve your health, not just the lab parameters, your cholesterol numbers must change on their own. They have to reflect your lifestyle habits, not the medication strength. Pill effect looks good on paper, but brings disappointing health results for the patient.

Chapter 6

Can the guidelines be wrong?

The value of total cholesterol as a screen for cardiovascular disease has been questioned many times. The argument is not recent and goes back to the 1950s when University of California medical scientist John Gofman discovered the LDL particle. After realizing that there are different types of cholesterol and that they play significantly different physiological roles, Gofman reported that total cholesterol is a "dangerously poor predictor" of heart disease [18] and should not be used for that purpose.

Gofman was intimately involved in cholesterol research and knew the ins and outs of its physiology. He warned doctors that the link between cholesterol and heart disease is more complex than previously thought and one cannot predict the cardiac risk merely by measuring cholesterol numbers. Unfortunately his cautions about overstating cholesterol role in heart disease were overshadowed by Ancel Keys theory claiming that fat kills.

Ancel Keys, a professor at the University of Minnesota, put forth the theory that fat was the cause of all cardiac misfortunes. As a regarded scholar he could not just state his belief. He had to prove his point with research. He accessed available studies and mortality tables and set himself on a mission to confirm that the correlation between fat consumption and cardiac deaths actually exists. He succeeded. Not only did his theory sound plausible, but he also made it provable.

He presented his findings to respected physicians who, after seeing Keys presentation, could not deny his sound logic. Keys charts were very conclusive and clearly demonstrated that deaths from heart disease were going up with fat intake. The presentation was very convincing. Fat and heart disease was now linked. From that day on fat got denounced as a danger to the heart.

But Keys cheated. He did not use all available data. He cherry-picked what fit well into this theory and what looked good on the chart. As an objective researcher he was supposed to use data from 22 countries, but he only used data from six. He did so because it was the only way to prove that fat kills. Factoring in all countries would have ruined his presentation.[19]

I am not sure about his motive. Was it to gain fame, or was it to gain fortune? None of that matters. What matters is the sequela of events afterwards. It is shocking to realize that it is Ancel's sneaky approach that is currently influencing your eating habits and your doctor's attitude towards cholesterol.

John Gofman's cried about the flaws of Ancel Keys' theory but nobody listened. The cholesterol hypothesis spread like a wildfire. It was eagerly propelled by profit-oriented food manufacturers, who saw gold in the emerging trend. "Heart-friendly" margarines, cholesterol-free corn oil, skim milk, and fat-free breakfast cereals went viral. Cholesterol was being ousted from the kitchens. In 1957 margarine outsold butter for the first time.

The war on cholesterol got a nod of approval from the government. In 1980 the US Department of Agriculture released the official statement *"eat less fat, saturated fat, and cholesterol"*. This statement was disseminated even though there wasn't any conclusive evidence that fat caused heart disease. Despite lacking definite proof the government moved to establish cholesterol guidelines. Even a strong warning coming from Japanese physicians that low cholesterol does not decrease, but actually *increases* the risk for strokes wasn`t sufficient to stop the snowballing trend against cholesterol. Starting 1986 blood cholesterol above 200 mg/dL (5.2 mmol/l) was no longer treated as a fun fact, but as a disease. [20]

The war on cholesterol continued even though a massive long-term study, published at that time, contradicted it. The Framingham Heart study, which followed 5,000 Massachusetts dwellers for several decades, demonstrated that people with declining cholesterol suffer premature deaths from cancer and heart disease when compared to those with steady or increasing cholesterol.

The Framingham study was a blow to the anti-cholesterol movement. If taken seriously it would have stopped profitable prospects of many food and drug producers. Its findings were truly inconvenient, especially that statins, cholesterol-lowering medications, were already selling and soybean oil dominated 70% of the market.

Framingham was not alone. Other studies defending cholesterol started to pop up. In 1999 a large Harvard study demonstrated that low saturated fat intake correlated with *increased* cancer risk. The findings did not matter, because someone's fingers were already too deep in the cookie jar. The health care industry spent US $263 million to lobby the US government in the first half of 2009 alone.[21]

In 2004 the *Journal of the American College of Cardiology* published yet another study undermining the cholesterol-is-a-killer theory. It strongly questioned the validity of measuring total cholesterol for the purpose of establishing cardiac risk.[22] The study demonstrated that mortality did not decrease, but actually *increased* when total cholesterol dipped below 180 mg/dL (4.7 mmol/l). The researchers also reminded that there is no evidence suggesting that women benefit from cholesterol-lowering therapies and such practices may actually be detrimental to the elderly. They also re-confirmed that lower cholesterol in elderly is associated with higher incidence of cancer and heart disease.

In 2012 Norwegian scientists chimed in with another study disarming the cholesterol theory. The paper published in the *Journal of Evaluation in Clinical Practice* strongly suggested that current clinical guidelines on cholesterol are not valid and need to be re-formulated. The authors pointed out many flaws that needed to be addressed urgently. Specifically they highlighted the following:

High cholesterol does not kill

Strangely, the opposite may be true. Cholesterol looks to be heart protective. It is a general belief that death toll from heart disease increases with increasing cholesterol, but that is not true. The correlation between cholesterol and deaths is not linear. It follows a "U-shape".

"U-shape" means that both the highest AND the lowest cholesterol numbers are bad for the heart that the heart prefers cholesterol somewhere in the middle. Interestingly, the *lowest* mortality from (ischemic) heart disease is not found at zero but at cholesterol levels *between* 193 mg/dL (5.0 mmol/l) *and* 270 mg/dL (7.0 mmol/l). These findings are in a stark contrast to the official health guidelines that demonize cholesterol levels above 200 mg/dL (5.2 mmol/l) and suggest, without exception, that the lower the better.

Cholesterol is good for women

Women seem to be protected by higher cholesterol. The authors of the study found that women with high cholesterol lived the longest and had fewest cardiovascular problems. An interesting conclusion, again contrasting the guidelines, was that moderately elevated cholesterol in women contributed to longer life and fewer deaths from heart disease.

There is a sweet spot for men

Just as it is in women, ultra-low cholesterol is counterproductive in men. Most men benefit from cholesterol between 193 mg/dL (5.0 mmol/l) and 228 mg/dL (5.9 mmol/l, because it correlates to fewest deaths. Cholesterol above or below this range increases risk of death from all causes. Current guidelines that suggest keeping cholesterol below 200 mg/dL (5.2 mmol/l) may actually put many men and women at higher risk of death.

Smoking does not always matter

Cholesterol levels above 212 mg/dL (5.5 mmol/l), when compared to even higher cholesterol levels, are not associated with increased risk of death regardless of smoking status. That means, smokers with high cholesterol have the same risk of death than non-smokers. In other words, once a person has higher cholesterol numbers, quitting smoking makes no difference to longevity.

Disregard total cholesterol numbers

Total cholesterol is a very poor estimate of cardiovascular risk and should not be used as such. The author stressed that the findings of the study *"contradict the popularized idea of positive, linear relationship between cholesterol and fatal disease. Guideline-based advice regarding cardiovascular disease prevention may thus be outdated and misleading"*.[23]

Despite strong evidence against cholesterol theory the official guidelines haven`t changed yet. They continue validating total cholesterol as a good screen for the heart and suggest that the lower the cholesterol the better the outcome. They contribute to the fear of cholesterol and mislead the public.

You may be scratching your head why would a guideline correction be such a difficult task. The answer is simple. The cholesterol-lowering business is very lucrative. The current value of cholesterol lowering drugs is estimated at US $29 billion[24] and lobbying is powerful.

Chapter 7

How good is low cholesterol?

I am yet to find a patient who would not be afraid of high cholesterol, a cardiologist that would not prescribe statins, and a health professional who would not cheer low cholesterol numbers. Everyone seems to be on a mission to destroy that fatty monster and keep it "under control." Everyone wants to keep it as low as possible even though the value of cholesterol suppression has been questioned by many independent researchers, who demonstrated that this common practice does not make things better for the heart and that lower cholesterol simply does not translate to fewer deaths.[25,26]

We got stuck. In our heads the cholesterol number 200 mg/dL (5.2 mmol/l) remains a dividing point between good and bad health. We want to stay below, never above. We seek out low-fat produce and zero-cholesterol goods just to satisfy that belief. We take natural cholesterol destroyers, and stuff ourselves with prescription meds in hope to please our doctors next lab test around.

But instead of promised benefits cholesterol-lowering practice maybe doing us more harm than good. Your doctor may not tell you that (he may not know it either), but low cholesterol not only does not deliver what it promises, but frequently leads to bad health.

Below is a compilation of various studies on low cholesterol. Although the presented studies may look similar to some readers, each actually provides a slightly different insight. The distinguishing details may not be important for an average reader, but they may present a significant value to those seeking increased clarity.

1. Low cholesterol does not prevent deaths

A detailed analysis of 22 studies revealed an unexpected finding. Lowering serum cholesterol would not make you live a day longer. Neither would it contribute to prevention of coronary heart disease.[27] This was the conclusion U. Ravnskov came up with after he investigated all controlled cholesterol trials.

Lack of positive results from lowering cholesterol may seem shocking considering that the whole medical system touts the opposite. Why would doctors continue the anti-cholesterol argument if studies prove it makes no difference?

Some insiders have an answer. Apparently such widespread finger-pointing is due to *preferential* citation of just a few anti-cholesterol trials.[28] Anti-cholesterol trials are six times more likely to be cited than pro-cholesterol or cholesterol-neutral tests. And that's how the cholesterol message gets skewed.

2. Low cholesterol increases chances of death from stroke

This is correct, even though practically every doctor claims the opposite. The general belief is that low cholesterol save lives. But you may want to think twice about lowering your numbers if you are concerned about major strokes.

According to several studies, deaths from strokes are inversely related to serum cholesterol. In plain langue it means that people with lower cholesterol have more strokes. This may sound strange and counter-intuitive, but people with higher cholesterol actually suffer fewer serious strokes and have fewer deaths because of them.[29]

3. Lower cholesterol increases risk of getting strokes

There are two main types of strokes: ischemic and hemorrhagic. Ischemic stroke is due to a clot. Hemorrhagic stroke, on the other hand, is due to a burst vessel. Ischemic stroke is most common in diabetics. Hemorrhagic stroke is most common in alcoholics.

These two different stroke types vary in mortality. They carry very different risk of death. Hemorrhagic stroke takes twice as many lives as compared to ischemic stroke. While only 25% people die from the first type, 49% die from the second.[30]

Cholesterol acts sort of like a clotting agent and thus safeguards against bleeding. Therefore, high cholesterol lowers the risk for bleeding strokes. The opposite is true as well. Lower cholesterol numbers increase the risk for hemorrhagic, the most deadly type of stroke. [31, 32]

4. Lower cholesterol prevents recovery from strokes

Lowering cholesterol has become a medical routine and its application knows very few exceptions. Such treatment is also suggested to patients that suffer strokes. However, recent research disagrees with such practice and suggests that lowering cholesterol may be counterproductive in these cases.

Studies show that lower cholesterol not only increases the risk for a bleeding stroke, but also prevents proper recovery after an ischemic stroke. They point out that lower cholesterol, does not increase, but actually *decreases* the chances for recovery after ischemic, the most common type of stroke.[33]

5. Lower cholesterol increases deaths in coronary artery cases

This link may turn out to be the most shocking. We are conditioned to think that higher cholesterol leads to atherosclerosis, blocked arteries, and eventually death, but this theory continues to be disproven.

Higher cholesterol does not cause blocked arteries or lead to deaths from lack of blood flow. It is low cholesterol that we should watch out for. According to *European Heart Journal* it is low, not high cholesterol that doctors should ogle, because cholesterol below 160 mg/dL (4.1 mmol/l) may be the most dangerous proposition for the heart.

This European study pointed out an unusual correlation. People with *low* total cholesterol have higher chances of dying from coronary heart disease than people with higher cholesterol.[34] Again, this is in complete contradiction to what health care professionals are being taught in schools.

6. Lower cholesterol does not prevent heart attacks

Many people lower their cholesterol in hope to avoid a heart attack, but this practice may not have any value. Heart attacks are most common in people with systemic inflammation and people with low *good* cholesterol. Total cholesterol numbers seem to have nothing to do with stopping the heart.

There are two groups of people who appear to be immune to heart attacks. According to the Framingham study one such group had ultra-low, the other had ultra-high cholesterol. Only these two groups, while being studied, managed to not suffer a single heart attack over several decades. What were these magic heart-saving cholesterol cut off numbers? One is below 150 mg/dL (3.9 mmol/l). The other is above 380mg/dL (9.8 mmol/l).[35] That's right. Heart attacks and cholesterol don't go together.

It is inflammation and low HDL that we should be afraid of. Reduction of systemic inflammation and increase of good cholesterol are the best safeguards against heart attacks. Lowering overall cholesterol numbers is ineffective and it does not translate to fewer heart attacks.[36]

7. Lower cholesterol worsens heart failure outcomes

Congestive heart failure is a severe condition. It causes fatigue, inability to exercise, swelling, and shortness of breath. As it is the case with strokes, heart failure patients should not run away from fats, because when the heart is congested and stalls the circulation, this is *not* the time to lower cholesterol.

Contrary to popular belief, congestive heart failure sufferers live longer when they carry *higher* cholesterol. The difference in mortality statistic is significant. As many as 92% patients with cholesterol *above* 200 mg/dL (5.2 mmol/l) manage to survive at least a year after the diagnosis. In comparison only 75% of those with cholesterol *below* that number stay alive past one year.

The current guidelines don't reflect these findings. Cholesterol above 200 mg/dL (5.2 mmol/l) is considered deadly for every adult. It does not matter that lower cholesterol puts congestive heart failure patients at higher risk.[37] The guidelines hold firm for everyone.

8. Lower cholesterol does not reduce arterial blockage

If you ever hear that high cholesterol clogs up arteries, know that this false claim is nothing more than an echo from Keys cheating days. Total cholesterol in the blood does not correlate with development of arterial streaks, which are responsible for initiating the process of arterial hardening.[38]

Since the development of atherosclerosis is not linked to total cholesterol, don't hope to clean your arteries by lowering cholesterol. Maybe it is now time to bring up the French paradox. Brits have four times more deaths from blocked arteries than Frenchmen. Yet, both have similar cholesterol.[39]

9. Lower cholesterol may shorten lifespan

Shall we fear high cholesterol and the deadly toll that follows? Maybe the margarine industry wants you to believe that but a 6-year study on elderly should put your mind at ease.

A Finnish study observed that seniors with the highest cholesterol lived the longest. Those with cholesterol above 230 mg/dL (6.0 mmol/l) far outlived those with cholesterol below 193 mg/dL (5.0 mmol/l) regardless of their health status.[40]

At least when it comes o a ripe old age, again contrary to the guidelines, one should be cheering rather than panicking about high cholesterol. Cholesterol may turn out to be one`s greatest longevity companion.

10. Lower cholesterol lowers testosterone

Since all steroid hormones need cholesterol there isn't any steroid that can be built without it. And that includes testosterone. Steroids are so dependent on cholesterol that cutting down its supply may stop hormone production altogether. Testosterone is not an exception.

So what happens to testosterone when cholesterol is short in supply? Scientists have the answer. Low cholesterol leads to lower testosterone.[41] Although not everyone's body responds the same, this finding should caution men wishing to remain manly. Testosterone is masculinizing and it is needed for gender-unambiguous sexual performance and male characteristics. Lowering cholesterol may not support this goal.

11. Lower cholesterol weakens immune system

The likelihood of developing cancer is astronomically high. It is one in two for all Americans.[42] Are we stuck to accept these terrible odds or is there a simple way to reduce them? It appears that keeping cholesterol up a notch may just be the answer.

Studies demonstrated that low cholesterol negatively affects the immune response. It has been observed that cholesterol numbers go down with infections. But why? Some suggest that cholesterol is used by the body when the immune system is challenged. [43] If this is true, then high cholesterol may be good for the immune system and low cholesterol may be reducing its power.

Cholesterol-immune system connection was studied in detail and indeed there is a meaningful correlation between the two. Low cholesterol can significantly lower immune system performance and increase the risk of death from infections as well as cancers.[44,45] Weakened immune system response is especially noted with total cholesterol below 160 mg/dL (4.1 mmol/l).

12. Lower cholesterol may increase cancer risk

Studies revealed that steady cholesterol, regardless of the actual numbers, is better than sudden fluctuations. Researchers warned that sudden dips of cholesterol should be very concerning. Its rapid reduction can herald a dramatic loss of health.

According to the analysis the most alarming were large cholesterol plunges of magnitude around 23 mg/dL (0.6 mmol/l). These were associated with risk of death within one year. Falling cholesterol has been mostly linked to cancers of the blood, esophagus, and prostate. Decreasing weight and decreasing cholesterol is a common finding in malignant diseases.[46]

But even steady low cholesterol may present a problem. A meta-analysis of 19 different studies came to the conclusion that people with cholesterol below 160 mg/dL (4.2 mmol/l) had higher chances of death than people with cholesterol between 160 mg/dL (4.2 mmol/l) and 200 mg/dL (5.2 mmol/l). A substantial proportion of these deaths were found to be cancer related.

13. Plunging cholesterol may herald bad health

Cholesterol is not just a cardiovascular marker. It is a health marker and its behaviour can predict wellbeing of a person. A 16 year-long study discovered that there is a strong link between plunging cholesterol numbers and development of some diseases.

The researchers found that a sudden decrease in numbers may precede clinical diagnosis of liver disease or cancer. While some diseases caused a tiny decrease, others cause a very large decline. For example, the largest drop was linked to esophageal cancer, the smallest to lung cancer.

Here are the drop magnitudes: esophageal cancer 22 mg/dL (0.57 mmol/l), liver disease 17 mg/dL (0.44 mmol/l), cancer of the blood 12 mg/dL (0.31 mmol/l), prostate cancer 15 mg/dL (0.39 mmol/l), rectal cancer 10 mg/dL (0.26 mmol/l), hemorrhagic stroke 3 mg/dL (0.08 mmol/l) and lung cancer 3 mg/dL (0.08 mmol/l).[47]

Periodic check of cholesterol numbers for non-cardiovascular purposes is highly advisable. Careful analysis of cholesterol behaviour can alert to a potential health decline. Artificially altered numbers do not offer such information.

14. Lower cholesterol is linked to depression

Did you know that low cholesterol and gloom go together? Did you know that people with lower cholesterol are more likely to be depressed, commit suicide, injure themselves or experience accidents and violent death?[48, 49, 50]

An 8 year-long study on 29 thousand people concluded that low cholesterol is linked to low mood and people with low cholesterol have a stronger need for emotional support and they are also more likely to require clinical intervention. All cardiologists should keep that correlation in mind and reconsider routine cholesterol-lowering practices in patients that are prone to depression as they may lead to serious consequences.

The above compilation of cholesterol studies hopefully sheds some light on the fact that lower cholesterol is falsely considered a universal health prescription and that is free of side effect. Cholesterol is the backbone of health. It is needed for proper function of neurotransmitters, hormones, immune system, muscles and even the heart.

It is chilling to realize that the highly popular cholesterol hypothesis relies not only on very weak data, but also on considerably distorted data.[51,52] Indeed, many studies, including the one published in *Annals of Nutrition & Metabolism in 2015* suggest that cholesterol plays a very positive role in health and should be treated as a friend, rather than an enemy.[53] And although treating lab numbers may be rewarding for the doctor, but it may not do the same for the patient.

Chapter 8

Don't bother going low-fat

Ok, if treating lab numbers for the sake of looking good is a bad idea maybe going on a low fat diet would translate to a better heart? After all, doctors and nutritionists must know something if they continue telling us to do so!

About 33% of Americans are on a diet and mostly the low-fat variety. DASH, Ornish, Cambridge, Slimfast, and other popular diets tell us that being heart-friendly basically boils down to trimming fat. But are low-fat diets as effective as advertised? Do they actually reward dieters by slimmer waist and lower cholesterol numbers?

Not really. 98% of dieters fail to lose weight and their cholesterol numbers seem firmly stuck despite their obsessive urge to trim the fat. This finding begs the question: is managing cholesterol such a difficult task or are we approaching the problem from the wrong angle? Surprisingly, the answer has been known to us for about a century.

Low-cholesterol diet effectiveness was debunked nearly a hundred years ago. In 1937 Columbia University biochemists David Rittenberg and Rudolph Schoenheimer clearly demonstrated that dietary cholesterol has very little effect on blood cholesterol. [54] Low fat diets are ineffective, because cholesterol is made in the liver according to the body's needs, not according to the number of eggs one has eaten.

Somehow this knowledge has crumbled under the pressure of profit-driven low-fat industry that managed to emphasize the importance of low fat diet despite studies suggesting that dietary cholesterol and heart disease have very little to do with each other. Even the government bowed under the low-fat pressure. Our health authorities stick to the idea that fat is bad and their health policies reflect this "truth".

Current official dietary guidelines are extremely fat-trimmed. Even though it is the liver that decides on blood cholesterol, health officials claim that we could manipulate our blood cholesterol at will by eating very little of it. Current guidelines for a heart prudent consumer restrict dietary cholesterol to less than 300 milligrams a day. That translates to about 1 egg yolk or 13 slices of cheese with zero-cholesterol foods for the rest of the day.

Since all animal products contain cholesterol after you've eaten your one-egg breakfast, you will have to abstain from pepperoni pizza, cold cuts, burgers, sausages, chilli, tacos, and even innocently looking baked chicken legs for the next 24 hours. Fortunately you have plenty of other healthy vegan choices. Since starches and carbs are cholesterol free you can satisfy the guidelines with a bucket of fries, coke, bread with jam, and two syrup glazed muffins on the side.

LOL, can you see the nonsense? Our health guidelines are so intelligent and smart. They make such health sense. Good luck to anyone who follows them. I myself decided not to act on this "expert" advice. You may follow me shortly, after reading how I eat and what cholesterol numbers I have.

I love fat and I have no intention of changing it. I don't pick low-fat cuts or spread my butter thin. I eat and eat well. My diet has about 2,000 milligrams of cholesterol a day. That's right. According to our health experts I should have a heart attack every morning because I start my day by exceeding the daily cholesterol guidelines. Yep, before the sun starts shining I sin by having 650% of daily cholesterol quota.

I eat about four eggs for breakfast. I put them on my organic toast that I grease with extra thick slices of organic butter. Yumm... This breakfast has about 1,500 milligrams of cholesterol, about five times more than I should have in a day. Health experts warn about such reckless behaviour. It can lead to high cholesterol and heart disease. Since I have been doing it for years, I should have some consequences by now. If not a stroke, at least I should succumb to obesity.

Despite all the warnings of an impending doom, my heart has never been happier. It ticks well and there is not a smidgen of misbehaviour. It beats 65 times a minute, works without a flutter and keeps blood pressure normal-low. And my cholesterol? Many cardiologists could get red jealous about the numbers. They indicate a superior cardiovascular health and squeaky clean arteries. How can that be? Do my eggs come without yolks? Has my butter been pressed out of its cholesterol? Am I on cholesterol-blocking pills? Nope. The guidelines have been, let's call it gently, "poorly formulated".

Here are my numbers after many years on high cholesterol menu:

TC (total chol) 158 mg/dL (4.08 mmol/l)

HDL (good chol) – 82 mg/dL (2.13 mmol/l)

LDL (bad chol) – 67 mg/dL (1.73 mmol/l)

Average blood **pressure**: 110/70 mmHg

Body **weight**: 128 lb

Age: 48

So what's wrong with the guidelines? Is it bad science, bad analysis, bureaucratic mistake, or just lobbying money at work? It is hard to tell. But one thing is sure. I am not the exception, neither my body came from another planet. I tested various diets on my patients and invariably confirmed that those who incorporate quality fats see pleasant surprises on their blood tests. Exactly the same butter-loving patients have the easiest time slimming down and keeping their cholesterol in perfect ratios. I am looking forward to the day when everyone drops the lies and agrees that it is not the fat that is killing America. It is processed food and sedentary lifestyle.

Until we realize that our demise has nothing do with butter and beef, obesity and heart disease will remain rampant. In 1910 when America used high quality butter lavishly, heart disease affected 10 percent of the population. Today it affects 45 percent despite massive preventative efforts and wide-spread health education.[55]

I am truly saddened about our dubious health stewardship. Low fat and low cholesterol meals are still recommended by the health agencies, clinicians, and nutritionists despite their uselessness. I think that they are not only pointless, but frankly dangerous.

Low fat diet may contribute to poor health and obesity

Low fat diets turn out not to be the best way to health. They neither produce a long-term weight reduction, nor do they help the heart. Low-fat diets are so ineffective that they do not reduce the risk of heart disease or stroke even in people who manage to lose weight or quit smoking.[56]

Several studies pointed out that low fat diets may not only be useless, but they actually may be contributing to ill-health. Due to their naturally higher glycemic value, low fat meals tend to promote insulin resistance and contribute to diabetes.

Note that since the low fat diet was introduced to the public, obesity has skyrocketed. In 1970s less than 20% of people were obese. Today, despite dietary efforts, obesity is close to 40%.[57]

Margarine contributes to poor health

Margarine became the "go to fat" for those who did not want to eat cholesterol. Since margarines are made of plant oils, they don't have any cholesterol in them. However, that does not make them heart-friendly. Many margarines carry compounds that aren't good for the heart. Although heart-killing hydrogenated oils, shortenings, and trans fats are now a rare find, many margarine brands continue being made of ingredients with doubtful reputation.

I encourage you to do your own product research. You may find that many types of "healthy" margarines you are told to eat, actually increase the risk for coronary artery disease. Interestingly, real butter doesn't.[58]

Eggs are safe

Cholesterol has been demonised as bad and so have the eggs that carry it. Your doctor may be restricting your egg intake in fear that it may impact your health. But the link between eggs and heart disease has been debunked a long time ago. Egg consumption neither increases cholesterol nor increases the risk for coronary artery disease.[59]

There is no need to be afraid. Eggs don't plug the arteries. They don't sneak out of the stomach and perfidiously squeeze themselves into the blood vessels. This fact has been known for over 30 years.

Butter builds health

Butter avoidance is a common practice among misguided health seekers. The logic is that butter, which carries cholesterol, blocks the arteries.

But just like eggs, butter is innocent. It has been wrongly accused of obstructing blood vessels. Current research suggests that butter is highly beneficial for the heart and also when consumed in considerable amounts.

Higher consumption of ghee (clarified butter) is not only associated with *lower* prevalence of coronary heart disease but also lower prevalence of liver disease, epilepsy, and memory decline. [60] Regardless whether you care for you heart, your liver, or your brain, I would suggest putting butter back on the table.

Being vegan is bad for the heart

Many people turn vegan to keep cardiovascular disease at bay. Unfortunately this is a false belief. Veganism leads to multiple nutritional deficiencies that not only cause health problems, but also directly weaken the cardiac muscle. Vegan diets are B12 and iron deficient and this leads to various undesirable health effects.

For example, lack of B12 leads to accumulation of homocysteine, a product which is directly toxic to blood vessels. Elevated homocysteine is an independent risk factor for developing of heart disease.[61] Lack of iron contributes to anemia, which reduces oxygen delivery to the heart.

Vitamin B12 and iron are not the only nutrients in question. Calcium, vitamin D and vitamin E are also frequently deficient in vegan diets, so is protein, creatine, and carnitine. These nutrients impact cardiovascular health either in a direct or indirect manner leading to various side effects. Calcium deficiency can cause hypertension. Vitamin E deficiency contributes to oxidative damage of blood vessels, and lack of carnitine can make the heart muscle inefficient.

What should you eat then?

If you want to have perfect cholesterol don't ever get sucked into the habit of dieting. Instead, make better meals your lifestyle mission. Multiple studies show that the strongest hearts co-exist with diets free of processed food and junk. And although such dietary practices do not lower cholesterol in a hurry they reduce heart attacks, strokes, and arterial plaque better than any man-made intervention.

Chapter 9

13 reasons to avoid statins

Sooner or later all heart conscious patients realize that low cholesterol diets fail. Some give up, some move into supplements. The disgruntled reach for red yeast extract, fish oil or garlic, only to be confronted by short term results. Those who keep up the pill taking habit may permanently trade their health dollar for stinky breath and a foul burp.

Lack of bullet-proof alternatives is exactly the reason why approximately half of Americans with high cholesterol are on lipid-lowering medication. What's easier than taking one pill that is guaranteed to work? Drugs perform well and they appear to make everyone happy. Lower numbers make doctors pleased and patients relieved.

But is this situation as win-win as it looks on the surface? After all, not addressing the causes behind high cholesterol and loads of side effects is not something we should call high standard. Besides not contributing to health, drug metabolites can be detrimental to the environment. They are, next to climate change, one of the biggest challenges we are facing today.

Even though the drugs can be harmful to both the patient and to the ecosystem many prescribing doctors downplay these concerns. They may be insisting that the drugs are safe and necessary, not because either is true, but because the drugs are their main, and frequently the only, tool to deal with heart disease. Standard medical training is insufficient to teach a doctor how to deal with cholesterol in any other way except reaching for his prescription pad.

The reality is that lowering cholesterol with statins is not as innocent as their prescribing laxity may suggest. Statins carry numerous adverse effects. Below are just a few of the negative effects discovered by research. Statins may:

Popular Statins:

- Simvastatin (Zocor, Simcard)
- Atorvastatin (Atrolip, Torvast))
- Pravastatin (Pravachol)
- Rosuvastatin (Crestor)
- Fluvastatin (Canef)
- Lovastatin (Altocor, Levacor)
- Pitavastatin (Livalo).

---

1. Accelerate hardening of the arteries [62, 63, 64]

This is not a joke. Exactly the medication that is supposed to keep the arteries clean has been found doing the opposite.

Although many lay people may be shocked by this finding, pharmacist should not be surprised. Such contradictory action is not unusual for pharmaceuticals.

There are many examples of paradoxical effect among drugs: cancer drugs can give cancer, antidepressants can cause suicides, and antibiotics can cause proliferation of superbugs. And thus cholesterol lowering medication can increase cholesterol buildup in the body.

Nobody knows for sure how statins do so, but there are some suggestions as to the reason. Statins block several vitamin K processes, which are necessary for keeping arteries clean. Vitamin K plays a very important role in blood flow. It reverses arterial calcification and prevents hardening of the arteries. When vitamin K is blocked, blood vessel elasticity becomes compromised.

2. Increase heart failure rate,[65] as well as mortality [66]

A study published in *Journal of the American College of Cardiology* raised a serious question about safety of statins in heart failure patients. The researchers followed two hundred patients that were prescribed statins as a prudent measure to reduce heart failure complications. The data was collected over several years.

The results were completely unexpected. Those with the lowest cholesterol had *the worst*, not the best outcome, and also had the highest death rate. Patients with total cholesterol levels below 200 mg/dL (5.2 mmol/l) were at 1.5 to 3 times the risk of dying as those with higher numbers.

The best outcomes were recorded for people with cholesterol *above* 200 mg/dL (5.2 mmol/l). These patients not only fared better, but they also had the lowest death rate. Researchers discovered a significant direct link between cholesterol and survival rate in heart failure patients. For each 40 mg/dL (1 mmol/l) increase in cholesterol, survival increased by 25%. This finding is in contrast to the guidelines that suggest keeping cholesterol *below* 200mg/dL (5.2 mmol/l) for everyone.

3. Increase rate of kidney failure [67]

Statins are not kind on the kidneys. Although kidney damage is a common theme for drugs excreted via urine, statins may be a tad more toxic to the kidneys than other common prescription medications.

A large 8-year study revealed that people taking statins were 30-36% more prone to kidney disease than those who did not take the drug. 43 thousand participants residing in San Antonio, TX were followed. 13 thousand of those were on statins for close to five years.

The comparison of the statin vs non-statin group revealed that patients on statins were more prone to both acute as well as chronic kidney failure. Kidney inflammation and kidney sclerosis (tissue hardening) were also 35% higher in the statin group. The authors of the study cautioned doctors about routine statin prescribing. They pointed out that deaths from kidney failure outnumbered the heart disease survival rates, statins were supposed to be responsible for.

4. Cause multiple nutritional deficiencies

No drug is free of side effects and many drugs contribute to malnutrition. Either they block nutrient absorption, cause difficulty in metabolism, deplete nutrient stores, or simply cause overuse of some nutrients. Statins are not any different.

Statins cause multiple nutrient deficiencies and they are most known for depletion of CoQ10. Ironically, CoQ10 depletion is detrimental to the heart. CoQ10 is essential for muscular contraction and since the heart is a muscle, lack of Co10Q causes cardiovascular havoc.

The heart muscle is extremely active and requires an uninterrupted supply of CoQ10 to function normally. Without CoQ10 the heart loses the power and stops pumping. CoQ10 cannot be replaced by other nutrients and its lack invariably leads to weakening of the heart. This is one of the reasons why heart failure patients don't do well with statins.

CoQ10 is not the only nutrient depleted by these drugs. Statins also contribute to deficiencies of other nutrients including selenium, zinc, copper, and various fatty acids.[68] These nutrients are essential for the function of multiple body systems including defenses and hormones.

5. Result in mitochondrial damage [69]

Mitochondria are the cellular power houses. These hidden tiny intracellular blobs seldom rest. They can't, because the cells rely on them to produce energy. Because of their role, mitochondria can be found in highly dynamic organs, such as the heart muscle.

Because statins are capable of impairing mitochondrial function, they can undermine health of the cells. If deterioration is substantial, whole organs or systems may start malfunctioning. Depletion of CoQ10 is at least partially responsible for the cellular energy shortage. However, because CoQ10 supplementation has not always been helpful, analysts speculate that there must be another mechanism that damages mitochondria besides CoQ10 deficiency.

Mitochondrial damage is especially problematic for elderly and athletes. These two groups rely heavily on muscles. While lacking physical strength can substantially reduce quality of life in elderly, in athletes it can halt the entire career progress.

6. Weaken muscles [70,71]

No one really knows what exactly statins do to mitochondria. Researchers can only speculate as to what happens inside the cell once the drug gets in. For now we only know that statins are capable of causing muscular weakness due to their mitochondria unfriendly attitude.

Not everyone reacts to statins in the same way. Some users may end up with myopathy, some with various symptoms. For some the symptoms may be limited to a minor ache, for others they may take the form of physical weakness. In unfortunate cases the problem can progress to myositis, a serious condition involving tissue inflammation.

Rarely, the usual cases of muscle inflammation progress to rhabdomyolysis, a life threatening condition characterised by very rapid destruction of muscle tissue. Rhabdomyolysis always necessitates an emergency treatment.

7. Cause memory loss, forgetfulness, and confusion [72]

Can you keep your thoughts together when cholesterol is in short supply? Let's say you will have difficulties. There is a reason why 25% of all body cholesterol is fixed in the brain.

Because of this tight brain-cholesterol connection, cholesterol shortage may lead to thought shortage, or at least to an altered mental state. This is exactly what happens to many statin users, who report that confusion and loss of memory appears shortly after starting the drugs.

Formal studies on the subject confirm such correlation. Any medication that lowers cholesterol, statin or not, can cause concerning mental side effects. Functional defects such as memory deficits, forgetfulness, and confusion are especially noted within the first 30 days of starting these drugs.

8. Increase risk for thyroid disease [73,74]

As it would not be enough that statins can damage the muscles or the mind, it appears that they can also produce changes in the other body parts.

A recent study revealed that statin users can also see hormonal alterations on their lab reports. It appears that statins are capable of modifying thyroid function or at least the lab numbers pertaining to the thyroid.

Statins can reduce TSH levels. TSH or thyroid stimulating hormone is a communicating molecule between the brain and the gland. Low TSH signifies either an insufficiency of the brain hormone or an excessive production of thyroid hormone by the thyroid. Either one is not healthy.

We don't have any plausible explanation for this phenomenon. Neither do we know what it means for the body. Some doctors point out a disturbing fact that the drug manufacturers continue to discover new side effects even though this class of drugs has been on the market for over 20 years.[75]

9. Can cause serious liver damage[76]

Statins work by blocking cholesterol production in the liver. But not all livers take such coercion lightly. Some do not tolerate being told what to do and fight back with inflammation. An increase in liver enzymes following statin regiment is common and that's why clinicians periodically do liver tests.

A recent Korean study[77] looked into liver enzymes with more detail. The authors noted that statin users were more likely to have increased numbers if they started with an already compromised liver. They also determined that liver damage was most likely to happen 3-4 months after starting the therapy.

Not all statins are created equal and some are more liver unfriendly than others. Korean researchers found that Atrovastatin was the least liver-friendly. It was implicated in 41% of elevated enzyme cases. Atrovastatin was followed closely by simvastatin, which affected 38% of cases.[78] Cholestasis, stagnation of bile, and damage to bile ducts were also reported, so were patient deaths due to acute liver failure.[79]

10. Damage nerves [80]

Cholesterol is essential for the function of the nerves. It gives them the ability to grow and regenerate. Without cholesterol the nervous system would slowly disintegrate. Studies confirmed that nerves cannot repair in a low-cholesterol environment.[81] This finding questions the practice of blocking cholesterol as a brain- and nerve-friendly treatment.

Every nerve fibre is insulated by a fatty sheet called myelin, which is vital to proper nerve function. Exactly that fatty envelope ensures an uninterrupted propagation of information along the fibre. Nerves without the myelin malfunction, scramble or lose the signal.

Statins interfere with building and repairing the sheet around the nerves. It is believed that the drugs do so by either providing a low-cholesterol environment or by interfering with the essential nerve-repair nutrients.

However, statins not only interfere with nerve regeneration or re-myelinisation. They are also capable of breaking down the existing myelin sheet, which makes them directly responsible for causing the nerve damage.[82] The problem is that such destruction may be carried on over a long period of time without any obvious signs to the victim. Many patients on statins do not perceive any symptoms, but studies confirmed a definite slowdown of nerve propagation after two years of drug use.[83]

The suspicion that statins cause accelerated muscle breakdown also emanated from the studies on marathon runners, that had much more extensive post-marathon tissue damage if they used the drug. The conclusion was based on analysing blood CK levels, an enzyme indicating the degree of muscle breakdown.[84]

11. Increase risk for type 2 diabetes [85]

The longer statins are on the market the more we become aware of their subtle, but potentially grave effects. One of the recently discovered concerns is that statins negatively impact blood sugar balance. Simply put, statins are linked to development of diabetes.

One study out of Finland reported that patients taking Zocor or Lipitor had 46% higher chance of developing diabetes than people who did not take these drugs.[86] Researchers believe that this side effect surfaces, because statins decrease insulin sensitivity and reduce insulin secretion.[87] Other studies find that statins also increase chances for diabetic complications and contribute to weight gain.[88]

Considering that diabetes is one of the major risk factor for heart disease one should seriously question statins as a genuine method for health improvement. Everyone knows that diabetes and healthy heart do not march in the same direction.

12. Increase risk for ALS and Parkinson's disease [89]

Amyotrophic Lateral Sclerosis (ALS) and Parkinson's disease are terrifying. They slowly turn a healthy person into a shadow of himself. The victim's body no longer can perform its functions. Nerves progressively malfunction making walking, swallowing, and breathing difficult. ALS patients eventually stop breathing, and Parkinson's patients either choke or fall down to their demise. The ugly twist to it is that the victim stays completely aware of his body deterioration but is totally defenseless.

Recently it came to light that statins may contribute to these diseases. There are more cases of Parkinson's disease in people taking statins than in those who do not. Also some cases of ALS have implicated statins as the probable disease catalyst.[90]

Since both ALS and Parkinson's are diseases of the nervous system it is not impossible to concede that statins, by reducing or depriving the body of cholesterol, can play a role in the appearance and acceleration of these diseases.

13. Prevent benefits of exercise [91]

Can statin side effects go as far as preventing one from excelling in sports? Despite patients' complaints about muscle weakness and nervous system misfires, statin manufacturers are adamant that the drugs do not change fitness parameters. They also claim that even though they change physiological parameters, statins do not change muscle strength or aerobic performance.

That however, seems to only be a partial truth. An independent analysis points out that statin manufacturers fail to mention that statin users do not improve their fitness parameters the same way as non-users do. VO2Max is one such example.

VO2Max is a measure of cardiovascular fitness. It estimates the maximum oxygen volume that a person can use. Oxygen utilization in turn determines the person's capacity to perform sustained exercise and is linked to aerobic endurance.

There is a drastic difference in athletic gains between people who take vs. those who do not take statins. According to the 2013 study published *The Journal of the American College of Cardiology*, 12 week supervised fitness program was sufficient to point out the obvious discrepancy. While non-users managed to increase their VO2Max by 10%, statin users only saw a 1.5% improvement. Some of them actually had their VO2Max lowered by the drugs.

How does exercise relate to heart health? According to statin manufacturers the drugs reduce heart attack risk by 10 to 20 percent for every drop of 40 mg/dL (1.0 mmol/l) in LDL levels. In contrast, regular exercise can reduce chances of dying from a heart attack by as much as 50 percent.[92] Exercise over statins?

Analysts also noted substantial discrepancies in weight and mitochondrial performance in these two fitness groups. Non-users lost on the average 1.7 pounds. Users actually gained weight despite following the same exercise regimen.

The biggest discrepancy however, was noted in mitochondrial markers. Non-users managed to improve their mitochondrial function by 13%, while statin group lost 4.5% mitochondrial power. Maybe it is worthwhile mentioning that a decline in mitochondrial energy is a major contributor to human aging?[93]

Chapter 10

I am confused, everybody says....

Strangely, when you do a Statin search on Google, you are likely going to stumble upon a litany of pages praising the drugs for their contribution to heart health. It would not matter whether you look at the first, second or third page. Page after page will state adamantly that you need to follow cholesterol guidelines and that statins are there to save your life. After reading the pages you surely will get convinced that statins are the unbeatable number one choice for ensuring safety of the heart. They reduce cholesterol, prevent plaque formation, reduce incidence of heart attacks, and prolong life. The claims are solid. They are backed up by official studies, the government, the medical establishments, and the media.

You are also likely to find pages with research stating that statin benefits extend way beyond cardiovascular system. Statins reduce inflammation, treat arthritis and even prevent Alzheimer's disease. The list of their benefits is very long and very convincing. Publicity works. Currently every third American over the age of 40 is on statins[94].

But are statins as good as the studies say? Many researchers disagree. After careful examination of all existing trials it turns out that statin benefits may have been overstated. Many statin trials were found to be flawed by reporting bias and a frank manipulation of data to overinflate their effects.[95]

A detailed analysis found that the manipulation techniques include

- purposefully terminating the trials to prevent exposing long-term effects
- under-reporting adverse events to show statins in their best light
- failing to mention a very high patient dropout rate due to side effects, and
- failing to admit of sponsorship by the very company that manufactures the drugs

Due to the above you would likely never stumble upon the information that nearly 75% of elderly stopped taking statins within the first two years due to side effects and 30% reported the primary cause for discontinuation was muscle pain and weakness.[96]

You may be shocked to learn that recent statin trials that followed new, stricter rules of reporting, failed to demonstrate a consistent mortality benefit, including elderly, patients with heart failure, patients with renal failure or diabetics.[97] Moreover, statins were found not to improve coronary calcium score as previously reported.[98] Coronary calcium score is a measure of arterial calcification and it is the most advanced way to measure arteriosclerotic lesions today.

Several researchers pointed out that the benefits of statins have been exaggerated and their benefit to harm ratio is so low that their routine prescribing should be questioned.[99,100] Some call statins an outright scam.[101] Many insiders point out that the actual decrease of mortality from cardiac causes is not due to statins, as the drug manufacturers claim, but due to other factors such as smoking cessation, lifestyle changes, improvement in hospital procedures, and use of defibrillators.[102]

Despite reporting bias, false advertising and lack of research transparency, statins are never better. In 2014 Americans filled out over 20 billion, or twenty thousand million, prescriptions for Crestor alone.[103] At US $7.11 per pill,[104] big pharma gets enough money to create unique content on thousands of Google pages.

Meanwhile it is becoming clearer and clearer that atherosclerosis is not linked to blood cholesterol, but to chronic inflammation and the cholesterol theory is nothing else but a big cash cow. We are discovering with astonishment that lowering cholesterol, with statins or other means, does not prolong lives and unless one makes positive lifestyle changes, there is little chance to stay healthy or live longer.

We are beginning to realize that cholesterol is not a killer, but a health marker which reflects the body state and function. It is an important messenger and a metabolic helper, wrongly accused of malicious behavior. We need to get it into our heads that cholesterol numbers don't go up and down randomly, but according to the body's needs. Cholesterol particles downregulate themselves into ideal zones after body health improves.

Do we even need to lower cholesterol or take statins to prevent heart disease? Statins could be praised for a 30% contribution towards decreasing cardiovascular mortality. Although this number may look impressive, when compared to lifestyle changes, the effect of statin starts to look meager at best.

A simple Mediterranean diet can decrease cardiac mortality by 70%. That's more than double of what drug manufacturers, after factoring in all their research techniques, can claim. But why didn't your doctor, pharmacist, or hundreds of pages on Google tell you that?

There are two simple reasons. First, the Mediterranean diet does not bring big bucks. The Mediterranean diet may be the best thing on earth for the heart, but as long as there is no profit to be made, no one cares to advocate for it.

Second, medical doctors lack training in nutrition to appreciate its value. Even though your physician may prefer self-care over prescriptions, and natural methods over chemical manipulation, he lacks training as to what, where, how much, and when.

There is no question that improvement in lifestyle habits brings much better results. [105] Neither there is any doubt that eating healthier is considerably cheaper than spending mega-dollars on life-long supply of prescription drugs. Lifestyle adjustments cost proverbial pennies. Exercise is free and food you have to buy anyhow.

Unfortunately the big pharma marketing strategy is so powerfully incentivised, so compelling and convincing, so precisely coordinated that neither care-givers nor patients themselves fathom to consider different options for their heart health. Pharmacological intervention pops up first in everyone's head even though drugs should be the very last choice.

Chapter 11

Cholesterol stories from the clinic

Cholesterol numbers are never random. There is always a reason why they decide to go out of whack. Reasons vary. It may be poor diet, inflammation, lack of physical conditioning, stress, nutritional deficiencies, chronic disease, adrenal malfunction, and many others.

The discovery of multi-causation became a huge turning point for me as a clinician and completely changed the way I started to treat cardiovascular diseases. Prescribing the same cholesterol-lowering regiment to everyone no longer made sense. Below I am sharing with you a few true stories of patients who were successfully treated with the new approach.

Emily

Emily was a 54-year old woman with good eating habits and a slim built, but her doctor insisted she needed to lower her cholesterol. She did not know how to go about it since she was already doing everything possible: she ate a healthy low fat diet, walked a lot and did yoga.

When I saw her blood work we had a long talk about her lifestyle habits. I ran some additional tests and made some conclusions. I told her that all her current efforts of lowering cholesterol were going in the wrong direction and instead of making things better, they were only contributing to her problem. She was shocked. She was following her doctor's recommendation. How can he be wrong?

It took her some time to understand the multi-causal concept behind high cholesterol and that standard dietary and exercise advice may not be right for her.

I walked her through her diet diary. Her diet was monotonous. It was based on whole grains, cereals and skim milk. She had skinless chicken breast and steamed rice for dinner. She had granola bars as snacks. She avoided butter, eggs, red meat, salt and sugar. When I asked why she eats like that she said that the menu was given to her by the doctor's dietitian as the most sensible means of cutting down cholesterol.

I told her to stop this low-fat nonsense, stop depriving and malnourishing herself. She needed to eat food, not processed shreds and instead, expand her food choices. I also told her she needed to have more variety, more soluble fibre, more animal products, and abandon glyphosate-sprayed cereals. I also advised her that walking and yoga weren't the exercise types her body needed.

She listened carefully and although while excited about new food choices, she was also extremely worried about the potential outcome. What if her cholesterol goes up, clogs up her arteries and kills her?

What if she ruins her health for good? What if her doctor scolds her for being a total fool?

She was confused by conflicting messages and hesitant about starting the new heretic approach, thus we agreed on a short-term three month trial. She was relieved to learn that if cholesterol climbs higher instead of going lower, she could always go back to her previous low-fat menu.

She committed herself. She abandoned walking and started jogging three times a week. She also brought variety into her diet and increased vegetables.

Two weeks into the program no one could deny the changes in her body. She was more energetic, happier, her skin got rosier, and she looked younger. Her neighbor, a medical doctor, stopped her a few times insisting that she could give away the secret to her youthfulness.

Three months later she repeated cholesterol tests. What a surprise! Her total cholesterol went down from 255mg/dL (6.59mmol/L) to 200 mg/dL (5.18 mmol/L) and her family practitioner completely stopped talking about statins. Instead, he asked her for advice. Specifically, he asked about the name of the natural product that was so effective. He admitted that he had a problem himself and did not want to be on drugs either.

Amit

Amit was a 73-year old Indian male with a litany of health problems: high cholesterol, obesity, gout, and chronic kidney failure. He was vegetarian and well set in his way of eating. He neither wanted to change his diet, nor was his family ready to accommodate it. In his world, culture and tradition was more important than the resulting health implications.

After the physical examination it became clear to me that Amit's excessive cholesterol was closely mirroring his excessive weight. Amit ate traditional Indian diet based on starchy vegetables, grains, and legumes, none of which he was willing to give up. A suggestion to reduce the calories through cutting down portions did not sit well with him either. I had to change strategy. I asked him to get a FitBit. Surprisingly, he liked that idea. He was an engineer and he liked numbers. He enjoyed mathematical analysis that came with the gadget.

Initially he wore it just so, to find out his activity baseline. After wearing FitBit for a week it became obvious that Amit is quite inactive, seldom making more than 2,000 steps a day and never peeking into the cardiovascular zone. Basically, I discovered he was sitting most of the time. He admitted he never exercised except his daily routine of slow yoga.

Lack of his cardiovascular effort did not matter at this moment. I did not plan for aerobic exercise to become part of his cholesterol prescription. His body was so unwell that any moderate or intense exertion would only aggravate his condition.

I explained the problem to Amit. The key was to make him lose weight without making changes to the diet. We agreed that an increase in activity is, in his case, necessary. We set the weight loss goal and made a few calculations. To lose one pound of belly fat in a week he needed to burn 500 calories daily through walking. He was open to it even though his gouty feet could present a major drawback. We decided that if his gout acts up he should aim for about 6,000 steps a day, and when his feet are fine he should aim for 15,000.

Three months later I got a new set of blood work from him. The cholesterol results were so altered that I suspected he could be on prescription drugs. I asked, but he said he wasn't on any pills. The only thing he did was faithfully making 10,000 steps a day.

Here are his before and after numbers

	Before	After 3 mo	Change
	mg/dL (mmol/l)	of 10,000 steps	
Total cholesterol	241.0 (6.2)	220.6 (5.7)	Lower by 9%
LDL (bad cholesterol)	161.3 (4.2)	122.0 (3.2)	Lower by 24%
HDL (good cholesterol)	39.7 (1.0)	57.7 (1.5)	Increased by 45%
Chol/HDL ratio	6.07	3.82	Lower by 37%
LDL/HDL ratio	4.06	2.12	Lower by 48%

If you are not sure how to interpret these changes here is a prompt: they are outstanding. They could be the source of envy for every patient and doctor aspiring to see better cholesterol numbers. And that's not everything. Amit lost 14 lb of stomach fat that was driving his cholesterol numbers up. His diabetes also started to reverse. He was very happy about the results and said he will continue. After all, he never considered being on pills. That felt unnatural. Walking was enjoyable.

Daniel

He was only 19 when I met him, but he did not look that young at all. He looked more like a man in his thirties at 5 feet 9 inches and 321 lb. Yet he was just between high school and college, stressing about the upcoming changes.

His biggest concern was that he would not be able to go through school because he had no energy and that his heart may give out. His medical doctor warned him about high blood pressure and high cholesterol. Daniel was lost. He was afraid to exercise due to his heart condition yet he was not willing to take blood pressure meds due to their side effects.

During his physical Daniel's blood pressure was high at 174/100 and his heart rate at 114, nearly doubled the norm. His cholesterol numbers were all over. Whatever was supposed to be low was high, and whatever was supposed to be high was low, indicating that the cardiovascular system in a serious crisis.

Additional blood work revealed that he was prediabetic, had low thyroid, and his liver enzymes were elevated. He had systemic inflammation, early stages of gout, and fatty liver.

It was already June and we only had two months left before he will have parted for college. We needed an intense program that would fit in Daniel's extremely busy schedule. Reorganizing his life wasn't an option, thus the program had to exclude dietary modifications or gym outings. Not that it mattered a lot, because Daniel's cholesterol was driven up mostly by stress.

I taught him a breathing technique that he would use daily and when he would feel nervous. He learnt re-focusing, visualization, and positive statements as additional coping strategies. I asked him to slightly cut down his meal portions and told him to take a few supplements. He ended up with a few antioxidants, a herbal concoction of choloretics, and a few basic minerals.

We repeated the tests just before he was headed for college. His cholesterol was down from 241 mg/dL (6.23 mmol/l) to 228 mg/dL (5.92 mmol/l) despite his daily eggs and bacon breakfasts. Triglycerides, which are considered an independent cardiovascular risk factor, also shrunk from high 87 mg/dL (2.27 mmol/l) to normal-low 37 mg/dL (0.97 mmol/l). Urate, a lab measure of gouty crystals, retracted to the normal range.

Although far from perfect Daniel's blood pressure started to calm down as well, averaging at 164/92. His heart rate hovered between 70 and 90, indicating better cardiovascular control. His weight loss was purely incredible. 41 pounds magically melted off him. With better heart and newly gained self-confidence he was ready for college.

These three stories may have inspired you to revisit your own approach toward cholesterol. You may even start questioning your doctor's prescription. However, before you decide to make changes, and especially, before you decide to go off statins be aware of possible consequences. Sudden cessation of statins is not free of side effects. Besides the fact that your cholesterol may go up uncontrollably, dropping statins can suddenly raise platelet count and make you more prone to strokes.

For that and many other reasons do not drop statins or any other medication suddenly or on your own. Find a knowledgeable physician that can help you with the transition. Your safety is the priority. Be smart. After all, you want to be healthier, not just drug-free.

Chapter 12

Let`s not kill the planet

The prospect of dying from heart disease doesn't make the future look attractive and the anti-cholesterol industry takes a full advantage of this scare. Fearful consumers are easy prey. The belief that low cholesterol equals health assurance drives them to try anything possible to get the numbers down, even if it means selling their soul to the devil.

I used to be part of the mainstream system. I used to lower cholesterol, because I was told to do so. But after having witnessed many patients getting heart attacks, strokes, and angina despite low cholesterol, I have drastically changed my approach on the subject.

Today I see things very differently. I believe that total cholesterol screening should be abandoned and cholesterol-lowering drugs should not be routinely prescribed. Total cholesterol is an outdated cardiac test and drugs often make matters worse. They not only carry side effects but they also prevent patients from making any lifestyle efforts. A vast majority of patients taking statins believe that low cholesterol numbers give them full amnesty from heart disease and that they will stay well no matter what. They don't bother making any lifestyle changes and frequently they become more sedentary and even more careless about their diets.

Besides not being of any help for people who need lifestyle adjustments, besides having many negative side effects, and besides draining the pocket, prescription drugs have yet another dark side to them, an anti-environmental attitude. Drugs pose a big threat to our ecosystem. We do not think about it, but massive quantities of drugs that get excreted by humans end up in our water and soil. Every time a user flushes the toilet he releases drug metabolites into the ecosystem.

There is very little media coverage about what happens to the drugs after we've used them. Shortage of publicity on the subject creates the naïve notion that drugs turn inert after being swallowed or that their remnants get filtered out by sewage facilities. Neither one is the case.

Drugs don't break down into nothingness, or water and air, as some may think. They break down to various metabolites that get ingested, inhaled, or absorbed by microbes, plankton, insects, fish, birds, mammals, and plants. We don't yet have the slightest idea as to what it means to the plants and animals, but the pioneering studies aren't appeasing. The amount of drug metabolites leaching into the waters is so vast that they no longer remain indifferent to aquatic life.

For example, clofibric acid, a metabolite of statins has been found accumulating in the environment in a rapid rate. Even in 1992 when lipid-lowering drugs were not so popular, clofibric acid was discovered in the ground water of Germany. Detailed studies revealed that at that time the North Sea contained approximately 150,000 lbs of clofibric acid, which is equivalent of 50-100 tons entering the sea every year.[106]

The spread of these chemicals is out of our control and the water purifying facilities are largely ineffective. Even before our pill popping culture flourished, drug metabolites flowed back to many homes via city pipelines. Such was the case in Berlin a few decades ago and things have gotten worse since then.

Today statins masquerade themselves as balsamic-glazed salmon fillets served for dinner. Lipitor together with Benedryl, Prozac, and Advil are now an integral part of fish meat, at least the fish caught in waters close to large cities.[107] We don't know yet what the consequences could be to fish or to humans that ingest the contaminated fish.[108] Currently we only know that statins act as herbicides and are toxic to plants living in water.[109]

We are running out of clean habitats. Even environments supposedly free from human meddling are saturated with pharmaceuticals. River estuaries that have no direct municipal treatment plant discharge are also mysteriously contaminated.

Pharmaceuticals pose a great risk to the entire ecosystem. Researchers warn that pharmaceutical residues leaking into the environment are capable of causing:

- Destruction of wildlife

- Unexpected mutations in animals
- Alteration of the environment and food sources for humans

For example, in India the entire population of vultures disappeared after they fed on cattle treated with the anti-inflammatory drug diclophenac. A diabetic drug, metformin, was found to be feminizing fish while decreasing chances for successful reproduction. Antibiotic by-products were found to inhibit plant growth and cause the development of drug-resistant bacteria[110]

Despite the magnitude, the problem seems to be escaping media attention. Pharma produces drugs, doctors prescribe them, and patients take them without either party being sufficiently concerned.

Our apathy and dis-concern in this matter is incredibly deep. The entire North American water supply seems to be contaminated by drug metabolites. Antidepressants, antibiotics, statins and hormones have been detected in 80% of streams and 93% of ground water in the USA.[111] In many areas ground water, tap water, surface water, and drinking water contains as many as 200 different drugs.[112] Lipid-lowering medication is just a fraction of this huge chemical pollution.

Our planet is no longer healthy. Humans have tampered with the ecosystem with devastating results. We are running out of sources of uncontaminated water and food. Our health, which is dependent on the planet's health, is declining. The need to change is urgent. It is time to deal with heart disease by addressing the causes, not the end effects.

Chapter 13

There is more than one way to bake a cake

Here is a simple, inexpensive, and environmentally-friendly plan. It targets the four strongest cholesterol-regulating life areas. These, when approached well, can give better results than the multi-billion dollar cholesterol lowering industry.

Don't be taken back by the simplicity of the plan. It is meant to be so. Exactly this ease can help every person and correct every lab report. And although the specifics of the personal plan must vary, rest assured that there are many different ways to have perfect cholesterol numbers while not getting stuck with expensive pills or unpalatable diets.

- **Eat well**. Say no to fast food and boxed food. Eat real food and put emphasis on variety, not on low fat.
- **Keep active**. If you haven't been moving a lot, aim for 10,000 steps a day. This is your healthy minimum.
- **Relax**. Don't take matters personally. If things regularly get out of control, consider learning better coping skills. Music is a great relaxant.

- **Relate**. Focus on building great relationships. Be honest, understand boundaries, and don`t hesitate to say no. Support people in need, be kind, and give hugs generously.

There is not one menu or exercise type that is better than the other. There is not one way to laugh or be merry. Whatever works for one person may not appeal to another. But don't worry. There is more than one way to bake a cake. Life presents a kaleidoscope of possibilities for every John and Jane walking on the planet.

So what are the best food and life choices for perfect cholesterol, longevity and happiness? Due to an incredible number of studies that I had collected I decided to reserve their presentation for another day. They will be gathered in a separate book on eco-friendly methods to escape the cardiovascular nightmare. No dieting, no pill, just skillful living.

For those who need just a little bit more direction today, here are a few examples of how to work the above plan into one's life.

- **Eat well** suggestions
    - Start your day with a glass of pure water
    - Add a tomato or avocado to your breakfast
    - Swap processed candy for real chocolate
- **Keep active** suggestions
    - Get yourself a wearable gadget
    - Walk with a buddy during lunch
    - Join dancing classes

- **Relax** suggestions
  - Fill your house with classical notes
  - Download binaural rhythms
  - Invest in deep breathing sessions now and then
- **Relate** suggestions
  - Get into a habit of smiling
  - Volunteer to help
  - Listen more than you talk

Make a short and sensible "to do" list that can fits neatly into your current lifestyle. Give it a try for three months and see what happens to your lab results, your weight, and your happiness index. Let your success lead you to an amazing discovery that Health is a Skill, not a Pill!

DrD

Cholesterol conversion chart

Mg/dL	Mmol/l
100	2.6
125	3.2
150	3.9
175	4.5
200	5.2
210	5.4
220	5.7
230	5.9
240	6.2
250	6.5
260	6.7
270	7.0
280	7.2
290	7.5
300	7.8
310	8.1
320	8.3

References

[1] Ross Toro, Infographic (2012). Retrieved October 28, 2016 from http://www.livescience.com/21213-leading-causes-of-death-in-the-u-s-since-1900-infographic.html

[2] Heart Disease Statistics, CarioSmart, *American College of Cardiology*. Retrieved October 28, 2016 from https://www.cardiosmart.org/Heart-Basics/CVD-Stats

[3] Heart Disease Facts, Centres for Disease Control and Prevention. Retrieved October 29, 2016 from http://www.cdc.gov/heartdisease/facts.htm

[4] Heart Disease and Stroke Statistics – At-a-Glance, American Heart Association. Retrieved October 29, 2016 from http://www.heart.org/idc/groups/ahamah-public/@wcm/@sop/@smd/documents/downloadable/ucm_470704.pdf

[5] Heart Disease Statistics, CarioSmart, *American College of Cardiology*. Retrieved October 28, 2016 from https://www.cardiosmart.org/Heart-Basics/CVD-Stats

[6] Cardiovascular Disease in the United States, Retrieved October 30, 2016 from https://sites.google.com/a/cornell.edu/cardiovascular-disease-in-the-united-states/

[7] Heart Disease Statistics, CarioSmart, *American College of Cardiology*. Retrieved October 28, 2016 from https://www.cardiosmart.org/Heart-Basics/CVD-Stats

[8] Overweight and Obesity Statistics, National Institute of Diabetes and Digestive and Kidney Diseases, Retrieved October 30, 2016 from https://www.niddk.nih.gov/health-information/health-statistics/Pages/overweight-obesity-statistics.aspx

[9] High Blood Pressure, Statistical Fact Sheet 2013 Update, American Heart Association. Retrieved October 30, 2016 from http://www.heart.org/idc/groups/heart-public/@wcm/@sop/@smd/documents/downloadable/ucm_319587.pdf

[10] High Cholesterol Facts, Centres for Disease Control and Prevention. Retrieved October 30, 2016 from http://www.cdc.gov/cholesterol/facts.htm

[11] Prevalence of tobacco consumption, Wikipedia. Retrieved October 30, 2016 from https://en.wikipedia.org/wiki/Prevalence_of_tobacco_consumption

[12] Facts & Statistics, American and Depression Association of America. Retrieved October 30, 2016 from https://www.adaa.org/about-adaa/press-room/facts-statistics

[13] Cholesterol metabolism. Retrieved October 30, 2016 from http://watcut.uwaterloo.ca/webnotes/Metabolism/cholesterolSignificance.html

[14] Forrest KY, Stuhldreher WL (2011). Prevalence and correlates of vitamin D deficiency in US adults, *Nutr Res. 2011 Jan;31(1):48-54.* doi: 10.1016/j.nutres.2010.12.001. PMID: 21310306. http://www.ncbi.nlm.nih.gov/pubmed/21310306

[15] Lindén V. (1975). Vitamin D and serum cholesterol, *Scand J Soc Med. 1975;3(2):83-5.* http://www.ncbi.nlm.nih.gov/pubmed/1179189

[16] David Perlmutter, Your Brain Needs Cholesterol, Retrieved October 20, 2016 from http://www.drperlmutter.com/brain-needs-cholesterol/

[17] G. Zuliani, M. Cavalieri, M. Galvani, S. Volpato, A. Cherubini, S. Bandinelli, A. M. Corsi, F. Lauretani, J. M. Guralnik, R. Fellin, L. Ferrucci (2010). Relationship Between Low Levels of High-Density Lipoprotein Cholesterol and Dementia in the Elderly. The InChianti Study, J Gerontol. *A Biol Sci Med Sci. 2010 May; 65A(5): 559–564.* PMC 2854885, doi: 10.1093/gerona/glq026. http://www.ncbi.nlm.nih.gov/pmc/articles/PMC2854885/

[18] Illustrated History Of Heart Disease 1825-2015. Retrieved October 21, 2016 from http://dietheartpublishing.com/diet-heart-timeline

[19] ibid

[20] ibid

[21] ibid

[22] Michael H. Criqui, Beatrice A. Golomb (2004). Low and lowered cholesterol and total mortality. *J Am Coll Cardiol. 2004;44(5):1009-1010.* doi:10.1016/j.jacc.2004.06.022. http://content.onlinejacc.org/article.aspx?articleid=1135936

[23] Halfdan Petursson, Johann A Sigurdsson, Calle Bengtsson, Tom I L Nilsen, Linn Getz (2012). Is the use of cholesterol in mortality risk algorithms in clinical guidelines valid? Ten years prospective data from the Norwegian HUNT 2 study. *J Eval Clin Pract. 2012 Feb; 18(1): 159–168.* PMC 3303886. doi: 10.1111/j.1365-2753.2011.01767.x http://www.ncbi.nlm.nih.gov/pmc/articles/PMC3303886/

[24] $29 Billion Reasons to Lie About Cholesterol. Retrieved October 16, 2016 from http://articles.mercola.com/sites/articles/archive/2012/02/01/29-billion-reasons-to-lie-about-cholesterol.aspx

[25] Eddie Vos, Colin P. Rose, Pierre Biron (2013). Why statins have failed to reduce mortality in just about anybody, *Journal of Clinical Lipidology, Vol. 7, Issue 3, pp 222–224.* doi: http://dx.doi.org/10.1016/j.jacl.2013.01.007. http://www.health-heart.org/Point-Counterpoint.pdf

[26] Mark H. Ebell (2014). Niacin Does Not Improve Clinical Outcomes in Patients

with Vascular Disease, *Am Fam Physician. 2014 Nov 1;90(9):660a-661.*
http://www.aafp.org/afp/2014/1101/p660a.html

[27] Ravnskov U. (1992). Cholesterol lowering trials in coronary heart disease: frequency of citation and outcome. *BMJ. 1992 Jul 4;305(6844):15-9.* PMC 1882525. http://www.ncbi.nlm.nih.gov/pubmed/1638188

[28] ibid

[29] Olsen TS, Christensen RH, Kammersgaard LP, Andersen KK (2007). Higher total serum cholesterol levels are associated with less severe strokes and lower all-cause mortality: ten-year follow-up of ischemic strokes in the Copenhagen Stroke Study. *Stroke. 2007 Oct;38(10):2646-51.* PMID: 17761907. doi:10.1161/strokeha.107.490292.
http://www.ncbi.nlm.nih.gov/pubmed/17761907

[30] Klaus Kaae Andersen, Tom Skyhøj Olsen, Christian Dehlendorff and Lars Peter Kammersgaard (2009). Hemorrhagic and Ischemic Strokes Compared; Stroke Severity, Mortality, and Risk Factors. *Stroke. 2009;40:2068-2072.*
http://dx.doi.org/10.1161/STROKEAHA.108.540112.
http://stroke.ahajournals.org/content/40/6/2068

[31] Okumura K, Iseki K, Wakugami K, Kimura Y, Muratani H, Ikemiya Y, Fukiyama K (1999). Low serum cholesterol as a risk factor for hemorrhagic stroke in men: a community-based mass screening in Okinawa, Japan. *Jpn Circ J. 1999 Jan;63(1):53-8.* PMID: 10084389.
http://www.ncbi.nlm.nih.gov/pubmed/10084389

[32] Iso H, Jacobs DR Jr, Wentworth D, Neaton JD, Cohen J.D. (1989). Serum cholesterol levels and six-year mortality from stroke in 350,977 men screened for the multiple risk factor intervention trial. *N Engl J Med. 1989 Apr 6;320(14):904-10.* PMID: 2619783. doi:10.1056/NEJM198904063201405.
http://www.ncbi.nlm.nih.gov/pubmed/2619783

[33] Vauthey C, de Freitas GR, van Melle G, Devuyst G, Bogousslavsky J.(2000). Better outcome after stroke with higher serum cholesterol levels. *Neurology. 2000 May 23;54(10):1944-9.* PMID: 10822434.
http://www.ncbi.nlm.nih.gov/pubmed/10822434

[34] S. Behar, E. Graff, H. Reicher-Reiss, V. Boyko, M. Benderly, A. Shotan, D. Brunner (1997). Low total cholesterol is associated with high total mortality in patients with coronary heart disease. *European Heart Journal (1997) 18, 52-5.*
https://eurheartj.oxfordjournals.org/content/ehj/18/1/52.full.pdf

[35] Robert DuBroff, Michel de Lorgeril (2015). Cholesterol confusion and statin controversy. *World J Cardiol. 2015 Jul 26; 7(7): 404–409.* PMCID: PMC4513492; doi: 10.4330/wjc.v7.i7.404;
https://www.ncbi.nlm.nih.gov/pmc/articles/PMC4513492/

[36] Haseeb A. Khan, Abdullah S. Alhomida, and Samia H. Sobki (2013). Lipid Profile

of Patients with Acute Myocardial Infarction and its Correlation with Systemic Inflammation. *Biomark Insights. 2013; 8: 1–7.* PMCID: PMC3561938; doi: 10.4137/BMI.S11015; http://www.ncbi.nlm.nih.gov/pmc/articles/PMC3561938/

[37] Rauchhaus M, Clark AL, Doehner W, Davos C, Bolger A, Sharma R, Coats AJ, Anker SD (2003). The relationship between cholesterol and survival in patients with chronic heart failure. *J Am Coll Cardiol. 2003 Dec 3;42(11):1933-40.* PMID: 14662255; http://www.ncbi.nlm.nih.gov/pubmed/14662255

[38] Cabin HS, Roberts WC (1982). Relation of serum total cholesterol and triglyceride levels to the amount and extent of coronary arterial narrowing by atherosclerotic plaque in coronary heart disease. Quantitative analysis of 2,037 five mm segments of 160 major epicardial coronary arteries in 40 necropsy patients. *Am J Med. 1982 Aug;73(2):227-34.* PMID: 7114080; http://www.ncbi.nlm.nih.gov/pubmed/7114080

[39] Malcolm Law, Nicholas Wald (1999). Why heart disease mortality is low in France: the time lag explanation. *BMJ. 1999 May 29; 318(7196): 1471–1480.* PMCID: PMC1115846; http://www.ncbi.nlm.nih.gov/pmc/articles/PMC1115846/

[40] Tuikkala P, Hartikainen S, Korhonen MJ, Lavikainen P, Kettunen R, Sulkava R, Enlund H (2010). Serum total cholesterol levels and all-cause mortality in a home-dwelling elderly population: a six-year follow-up. *Scand J Prim Health Care. 2010 Jun;28(2):121-7.* PMCID: PMC3442317; doi: 10.3109/02813432.2010.487371. http://www.ncbi.nlm.nih.gov/pubmed/20470020

[41] Kathleen Doheny (2010). Statins May Lower Testosterone, Libido. Retrieved October 21, 2016 from WebMD.com; http://www.webmd.com/erectile-dysfunction/news/20100416/statins_may_lower_testosterone_libido

[42] Lifetime Probability of Developing* and Dying from Cancer for 23 Sites, 2010-2012. American Cancer Society, Surveillance Research, 2016. Retrieved October 28, 2016 from Cancer.org; http://www.cancer.org/acs/groups/content/@research/documents/document/acspc-047075.pdf

[43] David R. Jacobs, Jr., Brian Hebert, Pamela J. Schreiner, Stephen Sidney, Carlos Iribarren, Stephen Hulley (1997). Reduced Cholesterol Is Associated with Recent Minor Illness. *American Journal of Epidemiology, Vol. 146, No. 7.* http://aje.oxfordjournals.org/content/146/7/558.full.pdf

[44] Elaine N. Meilahn (1995). Low Serum Cholesterol Hazardous to Health? *Circulation. 1995;92:2365-2366.* http://dx.doi.org/10.1161/01.CIR.92.9.2365; http://circ.ahajournals.org/content/92/9/2365

[45] Yun-Mi Song, Joohon Sung, Joung Soon Kim (1998). Which Cholesterol Level Is

Related to the Lowest Mortality in Population with Low Mean Cholesterol Level: A 6.4-Year Follow-up Study of 482,472 Korean Men. *American Jnl of Epidemiology Volume 151, Issue 8Pp. 739-747.* http://aje.oxfordjournals.org/content/151/8/739

[46] Elaine N. Meilahn (1995). Low Serum Cholesterol Hazardous to Health? *Circulation. 1995;92:2365-2366.* http://dx.doi.org/10.1161/01.CIR.92.9.2365; http://circ.ahajournals.org/content/92/9/2365

[47] Carlos Iribarren, Dwayne M. Reed, Randi Chen, Katsuhiko Yano and James H. Dwyer (1995). Low Serum Cholesterol and Mortality. Which Is the Cause and Which Is the Effect? *Circulation. 1995;92:2396-2403.* http://dx.doi.org/10.1161/01.CIR.92.9.2396; http://circ.ahajournals.org/content/92/9/2396

[48] Elaine N. Meilahn (1995). Low Serum Cholesterol Hazardous to Health? *Circulation. 1995;92:2365-2366.* http://dx.doi.org/10.1161/01.CIR.92.9.2365; http://circ.ahajournals.org/content/92/9/2365

[49] James M. Greenblatt M.D. (2011). Low Cholesterol and Its Psychological Effects. Retrieved August 11,2016 from Psychologytoday.com. https://www.psychologytoday.com/blog/the-breakthrough-depression-solution/201106/low-cholesterol-and-its-psychological-effects

[50] Partonen T, Haukka J, Virtamo J, Taylor PR, Lönnqvist J. (1999). Association of low serum total cholesterol with major depression and suicide. *Br J Psychiatry. 1999 Sep;175:259-62.* PMID: 10645328; http://www.ncbi.nlm.nih.gov/pubmed/10645328

[51] Chart: Total cholesterol levels vs mortality data from 164 COUNTRIES Retrieved November 1, 2016 from http://biohackyourself.com/wp-content/uploads/2013/01/Mortality-v-Chol1.pdf

[52] S. Karger AG (2015). *Ann Nutr Metab 2015;66(suppl 4):1–116.* doi: 10.1159/000381654; https://www.karger.com/Article/Pdf/381654

[53] ibid

[54] Illustrated History Of Heart Disease 1825-2015. Retrieved October 21, 2016 from http://dietheartpublishing.com/diet-heart-timeline

[55] ibid

[56] https://www.nih.gov/news-events/news-releases/news-womens-health-initiative-reducing-total-fat-intake-may-have-small-effect-risk-breast-cancer-no-effect-risk-colorectal-cancer-heart-disease-or-stroke

[57] Kris Gunnars. Do Low-Fat Diets Actually Work? A Critical Look. Retrieved October 30, 2016 from https://authoritynutrition.com/do-low-fat-diets-work/

[58] Gillman MW, Cupples LA, Gagnon D, Millen BE, Ellison RC, Castelli WP. (1997). Margarine intake and subsequent coronary heart disease in men. *Epidemiology. 1997 Mar;8(2):144-9.* PMID: 9229205;

http://www.ncbi.nlm.nih.gov/pubmed/9229205

[59] Dawber TR, Nickerson RJ, Brand FN, Pool J. (1982). Eggs, serum cholesterol, and coronary heart disease. *Am J Clin Nutr. 1982 Oct;36(4):617-25.* PMID: 7124663; http://www.ncbi.nlm.nih.gov/pubmed/7124663

[60] Hari Sharma, Xiaoying Zhang, and Chandradhar Dwivedi (2010). The effect of ghee (clarified butter) on serum lipid levels and microsomal lipid peroxidation. *Ayu. 2010 Apr-Jun; 31(2): 134–140.* PMCID: PMC3215354; doi: 10.4103/0974-8520.72361; http://www.ncbi.nlm.nih.gov/pmc/articles/PMC3215354/

[61] Paul Ganguly, Sreyoshi Fatima Alam (2015). Role of homocysteine in the development of cardiovascular disease. *Nutr J. 2015; 14: 6.* PMCID: PMC4326479; doi: 10.1186/1475-2891-14-6; https://www.ncbi.nlm.nih.gov/pmc/articles/PMC4326479/

[62] Okuyama H, Langsjoen PH, Ohara N, Hashimoto Y, Hamazaki T, Yoshida S, Kobayashi T, Langsjoen AM *(2016).* Medicines and Vegetable Oils as Hidden Causes of Cardiovascular Disease and Diabetes. *Pharmacology. 2016;98(3-4):134-70.* PMID: 27251151; doi: 10.1159/000446704. http://www.ncbi.nlm.nih.gov/pubmed/27251151

[63] Okuyama H, Langsjoen PH, Hamazaki T, Ogushi Y, Hama R, Kobayashi T, Uchino H.(2015). Statins stimulate atherosclerosis and heart failure: pharmacological mechanisms. *Expert Rev Clin Pharmacol. 2015 Mar;8(2):189-99.* PMID: 25655639; doi: 10.1586/17512433.2015.1011125; http://www.ncbi.nlm.nih.gov/pubmed/25655639

[64] ibid

[65] Okuyama H, Langsjoen PH, Ohara N, Hashimoto Y, Hamazaki T, Yoshida S, Kobayashi T, Langsjoen AM *(2016).* Medicines and Vegetable Oils as Hidden Causes of Cardiovascular Disease and Diabetes. *Pharmacology. 2016;98(3-4):134-70.* PMID: 27251151; doi: 10.1159/000446704. http://www.ncbi.nlm.nih.gov/pubmed/27251151

[66] Gregg C Fonarow, Tamara B Horwich (2003). Cholesterol and mortality in heart failure: the bad gone good? *Journal of the American College of Cardiology Volume 42, Issue 11, December 2003. doi:* 10.1016/j.jacc.2003.09.005; http://content.onlinejacc.org/article.aspx?articleid=1132834

[67] Marlene Busko (2015). More Kidney Disease With Long-Term Statins Seen in Cohort Study. Retrieved October 26, from Medscape.com; http://www.medscape.com/viewarticle/856244

[68] Alan Simon. Drug-Induced Nutrient Depletions. Retrieved November 12th 2016 from IntegrativeRxPharmacy.com http://integrativerxpharmacy.com/drug-induced%20nutrient040709b.pdf

[69] Richard Deichmann, MD, Carl Lavie, MD, and Samuel Andrews, MD (2010). Coenzyme Q10 and Statin-Induced Mitochondrial Dysfunction. *Ochsner J. 2010*

Spring; 10(1): 16–21. PMCID: PMC3096178;
http://www.ncbi.nlm.nih.gov/pmc/articles/PMC3096178/

[70] Beth A. Parker, Paul D. Thompson (2013). Effect of Statins on Skeletal Muscle: Exercise, Myopathy, and Muscle Outcomes. *Exerc Sport Sci Rev. 2012 Oct; 40(4): 188–194.* PMCID: PMC3463373; doi: 10.1097/JES.0b013e31826c169e; http://www.ncbi.nlm.nih.gov/pmc/articles/PMC3463373/

[71] Side Effects of Cholesterol-Lowering Statin Drugs. Retrieved October 3, 2016 from WebMD.com http://www.webmd.com/cholesterol-management/side-effects-of-statin-drugs?page=2

[72] Strom BL, Schinnar R, Karlawish J, Hennessy S, Teal V, Bilker WB. (2015). Statin Therapy and Risk of Acute Memory Impairment. *JAMA Intern Med. 2015 Aug;175(8):1399-405.* PMID: 26054031; doi: 10.1001/jamainternmed.2015.2092; http://www.ncbi.nlm.nih.gov/pubmed/26054031

[73] Beatrice A. Golomb, Marcella A. Evans (2008). Statin Adverse Effects: A Review of the Literature and Evidence for a Mitochondrial Mechanism. *Am J Cardiovasc Drugs. Am J Cardiovasc Drugs. 2008; 8(6): 373–418.* PMCID: PMC2849981; http://www.ncbi.nlm.nih.gov/pmc/articles/PMC2849981/

[74] Gouton M.(1993). Hypothyroidism, hypocholesteremic agents and rhabdomyolysis. *Arch Mal Coeur Vaiss. 1993 Dec;86(12):1761-4.* PMID: 8024378; https://www.ncbi.nlm.nih.gov/pubmed/8024378

[75] Duane Graveline, Abnormal Thyroid Function with Statins. Retrieved October 13, 2016 from https://www.spacedoc.com/articles/thyroid-and-statins

[76] Mayo Clinic Staff. Statin side effects: Weigh the benefits and risks. Retrieved October 11, 2016 from MayoClinic.org; http://www.mayoclinic.org/diseases-conditions/high-blood-cholesterol/in-depth/statin-side-effects/art-20046013

[77] Kim HS, Lee SH, Kim H, Lee SH, Cho JH, Lee H, Yim HW, Kim SH, Choi IY, Yoon KH, Kim JH (2016). Statin-related aminotransferase elevation according to baseline aminotransferases level in real practice in Korea. *J Clin Pharm Ther. 2016 Jun;41(3):266-72.* doi: 10.1111/jcpt.12377. PMID: 27015878; https://www.ncbi.nlm.nih.gov/pubmed/27015878

[78] Björnsson E, Jacobsen EI, Kalaitzakis E (2012). Hepatotoxicity associated with statins: reports of idiosyncratic liver injury post-marketing. *J Hepatol. 2012 Feb;56(2):374-80.* PMID: 21889469; doi: 10.1016/j.jhep.2011.07.023. https://www.ncbi.nlm.nih.gov/pubmed/21889469

[79] Rahier JF, Rahier J, Leclercq I, Geubel AP (2008). Severe acute cholestatic hepatitis with prolonged cholestasis and bile-duct injury following atorvastatin therapy: a case report. *Acta Gastroenterol Belg. 2008 Jul-Sep;71(3):318-20.* PMID: 19198578; .https://www.ncbi.nlm.nih.gov/pubmed/19198578

[80] Mayo Clinic Staff. Statin side effects: Weigh the benefits and risks. Retrieved

October 11, 2016 from MayoClinic.org; http://www.mayoclinic.org/diseases-conditions/high-blood-cholesterol/in-depth/statin-side-effects/art-20046013

[81] Saher G, Brügger B, Lappe-Siefke C, Möbius W, Tozawa R, Wehr MC, Wieland F, Ishibashi S, Nave KA. (2005). High cholesterol level is essential for myelin membrane growth. *Nat Neurosci. 2005 Apr;8(4):468-75. Epub 2005 Mar 27.* PMID: 15793579; doi: 10.1038/nn1426; https://www.ncbi.nlm.nih.gov/pubmed/15793579

[82] Tierney EF, Thurman DJ, Beckles GL, Cadwell BL (2013). Association of statin use with peripheral neuropathy in the U.S. population 40 years of age or older. *J Diabetes. 2013 Jun;5(2):207-15.* PMID: 23121724; doi: 10.1111/1753-0407.12013; . https://www.ncbi.nlm.nih.gov/pubmed/23121724

[83] Otruba P, Kanovsky P, Hlustik P (2011). Treatment with statins and peripheral neuropathy: results of 36-months a prospective clinical and neurophysiological follow-up. *Neuro Endocrinol Lett. 2011;32(5):688-90.* PMID: 22167150; https://www.ncbi.nlm.nih.gov/pubmed/22167150

[84] Beth A. Parker, Paul D. Thompson (2013). Effect of Statins on Skeletal Muscle: Exercise, Myopathy, and Muscle Outcomes. *Exerc Sport Sci Rev. 2012 Oct; 40(4): 188–194.* PMCID: PMC3463373; doi: 10.1097/JES.0b013e31826c169e; http://www.ncbi.nlm.nih.gov/pmc/articles/PMC3463373/

[85] Lipitor and Type 2 Diabetes. Retrieved October 26, 2016 from DrugWatch.com; https://www.drugwatch.com/lipitor/diabetes/

[86] Statins Side Effects - Diabetes, Rhabdomyolysis & Cardiomyopathy. Retrieved October 26, 2016 from LawyerAndSettlements.com; https://www.lawyersandsettlements.com/lawsuit/statins.html

[87] Cederberg H, Stančáková A, Yaluri N, Modi S, Kuusisto J, Laakso M. (2015). Increased risk of diabetes with statin treatment is associated with impaired insulin sensitivity and insulin secretion: a 6 year follow-up study of the METSIM cohort. *Diabetologia. 2015 May;58(5):1109-17.* PMID: 25754552; doi: 10.1007/s00125-015-3528-5. https://www.ncbi.nlm.nih.gov/pubmed/25754552

[88] Mansi I, Frei CR, Wang CP, Mortensen EM (2015). Statins and New-Onset Diabetes Mellitus and Diabetic Complications: A Retrospective Cohort Study of US Healthy Adults. *J Gen Intern Med. 2015 Nov;30(11):1599-610.* doi: 10.1007/s11606-015-3335-1. PMCID: PMC4617949; https://www.ncbi.nlm.nih.gov/pubmed/25917657

[89] Huang X, Alonso A, Guo X, Umbach DM, Lichtenstein ML, Ballantyne CM, Mailman RB, Mosley TH, Chen H (2015). Statins, plasma cholesterol, and risk of Parkinson's disease: a prospective study. *Mov Disord. 2015 Apr;30(4):552-9.* PMCID: PMC4390443; doi: 10.1002/mds.26152. Epub 2015 Jan 14. http://www.ncbi.nlm.nih.gov/pubmed/25639598

[90] Duane Graveline, ALS and Statins. Retrieved October 24, 2016 from https://www.spacedoc.com/articles/als-and-statins

[91] Statins prevent exercise benefits. Retrieved October 16, 2016 from http://n2shape.com/statins-prevent-exercise-benefits/

[92] ibid

[93] Lee HC, Wei YH.(2012). Mitochondria and aging. *Adv Exp Med Biol. 2012;942:311-27.* PMID: 22399429; doi: 10.1007/978-94-007-2869-1_14. https://www.ncbi.nlm.nih.gov/pubmed/22399429

[94] Steven Reinberg (2014). Number of Americans Taking Statins Keeps Rising: CDC. Retrieved 24th September, 2016 from https://consumer.healthday.com/general-health-information-16/misc-drugs-news-218/number-of-americans-taking-statins-keeps-rising-cdc-694895.html

[95] David M Diamond (2015). How statistical deception created the appearance that statins are safe and effective in primary and secondary prevention of cardiovascular disease. *Journal Expert Review of Clinical Pharmacology Volume 8, 2015 – Issue 2. pp201-210.* http://dx.doi.org/10.1586/17512433.2015.1012494; http://www.tandfonline.com/doi/abs/10.1586/17512433.2015.1012494

[96] Robert DuBroff, Michel de Lorgeril (2015). Cholesterol confusion and statin controversy. *World J Cardiol. 2015 Jul 26; 7(7): 404–409.* PMCID: PMC4513492; doi: 10.4330/wjc.v7.i7.404; https://www.ncbi.nlm.nih.gov/pmc/articles/PMC4513492/

[97] ibid

[98] Gill EA Jr (2010). Does statin therapy affect the progression of atherosclerosis measured by a coronary calcium score? *Curr Atheroscler Rep. 2010 Mar;12(2):83-7.* PMID: 20425242; doi: 10.1007/s11883-009-0073-z. https://www.ncbi.nlm.nih.gov/pubmed/20425242

[99] S. Karger AG (2015). *Ann Nutr Metab 2015;66(suppl 4):1–116.* doi: 10.1159/000381654; https://www.karger.com/Article/Pdf/381654

[100] Robert DuBroff, Michel de Lorgeril (2015). Cholesterol confusion and statin controversy. *World J Cardiol. 2015 Jul 26; 7(7): 404–409.* PMCID: PMC4513492; doi: 10.4330/wjc.v7.i7.404; https://www.ncbi.nlm.nih.gov/pmc/articles/PMC4513492/

[101] Paul Fassa (2016). Statin Scam and the Cholesterol Myth: Know the Truth. Retrieved September 22nd, 2016 from https://healthimpactnews.com/2016/statin-scam-and-the-cholesterol-myth-know-the-truth/

[102] Robert DuBroff, Michel de Lorgeril (2015). Cholesterol confusion and statin controversy. *World J Cardiol. 2015 Jul 26; 7(7): 404–409.* PMCID: PMC4513492; doi: 10.4330/wjc.v7.i7.404;

https://www.ncbi.nlm.nih.gov/pmc/articles/PMC4513492/

[103] Troy Brown (2015). 100 Best-Selling, Most Prescribed Branded Drugs Through March. Retrieved September 29th 2016 from MedScape.com http://www.medscape.com/viewarticle/844317

[104] http://www.moneycrashers.com/cost-most-prescribed-drugs-dont-need/

[105] Robert DuBroff, Michel de Lorgeril (2015). Cholesterol confusion and statin controversy. *World J Cardiol. 2015 Jul 26; 7(7): 404–409.* PMCID: PMC4513492; doi: 10.4330/wjc.v7.i7.404; https://www.ncbi.nlm.nih.gov/pmc/articles/PMC4513492/

[106] Bradford S. Weeks (2012). Statins polluting the environment. Retrieved October 2, 2016 from WeeksMD.com; http://weeksmd.com/2012/05/statins-polluting-the-environment/

[107] Eric Chaney (2016). Salmon Caught Near Seattle Test Positive For Wide Range of Drugs. Retrieved November 17th, 2016 from TheWeather.com https://weather.com/news/news/salmon-caught-near-seattle-tested-positive-for-wide-range-of-drugs

[108] Alistair B.A. Boxall (2004). The environmental side effects of medication. Table 2: Reported subtle effects of pharmaceutical compounds on aquatic and terrestrial organisms. *EMBO Rep. 2004 Dec; 5(12): 1110–1116.* PMCID: PMC1299201; http://www.ncbi.nlm.nih.gov/pmc/articles/PMC1299201/table/t2/

[109] Richard A. Brain, Tamara S. Reitsma, Linda I. Lissemore , Ketut (Jim) Bestari , Paul K. Sibley , Keith R. Solomon (2006). Herbicidal Effects of Statin Pharmaceuticals in Lemna gibba. *Environ. Sci. Technol., 2006, 40 (16), pp 5116–5123.* doi: 10.1021/es0600274; http://pubs.acs.org/doi/pdf/10.1021/es0600274

[110] Frank-Andreas Weber, Tim aus der Beek, Axel Bergmann, Alexander Carius, Gregor Grüttner, Silke Hickmann, Ina Ebert, Arne Hein, Anette Küster, Johanna Rose, Juliane Koch-Jugl, Hans-Christian Stolzenberg (2014). Pharmaceuticals in the environment – the global perspective. German Federal Environmental Agency. https://www.umweltbundesamt.de/sites/default/files/medien/378/publikationen/pharmaceuticals_in_the_environment_0.pdf

[111] Kevin Meehan (2014). The Effect of Medications on the Environment. Retrieved October 25, 2016 from MeehanFormulations.com; http://www.meehanformulations.com/blogs/articles/14137897-the-effect-of-medications-on-the-environment

[112] Frank-Andreas Weber, Tim aus der Beek, Axel Bergmann, Alexander Carius, Gregor Grüttner, Silke Hickmann, Ina Ebert, Arne Hein, Anette Küster, Johanna Rose, Juliane Koch-Jugl, Hans-Christian Stolzenberg (2014). Pharmaceuticals in

the environment – the global perspective. German Federal Environmental Agency. https://www.umweltbundesamt.de/sites/default/files/medien/378/publikatio nen/pharmaceuticals_in_the_environment_0.pdf